100 DELICIOUSLY
FUN & EASY
RAW VEGAN RECIPES

GLUTEN-FREE | OIL-FREE
NO DEHYDRATOR REQUIRED

JEANNETTE DONOFRIO

YOU ARE **THE MOST** IMPORTANT PERSON
IN YOUR LIFE

AND WITHOUT YOUR HEALTH...
YOU HAVE NOTHING!

THANK YOU FOR INVESTING
IN YOURSELF!

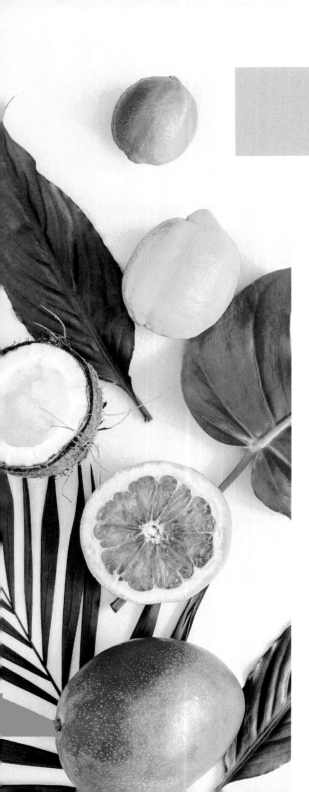

CONTENTS

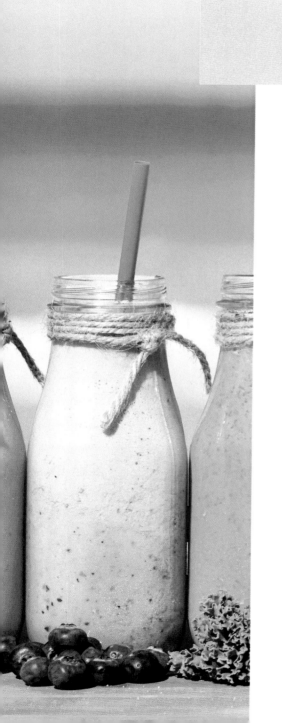

CONTENTS
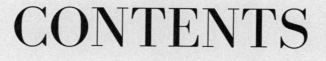

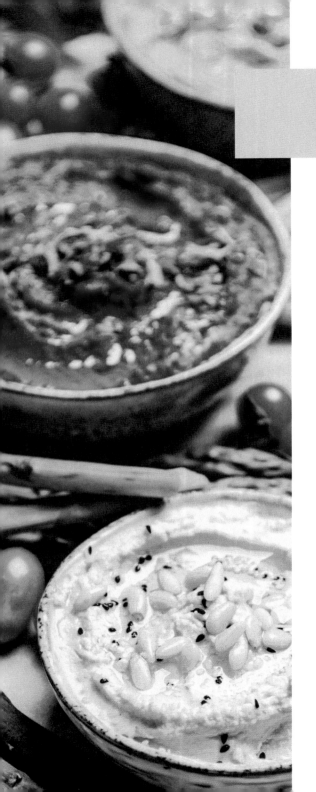

CONTENTS

DINNER

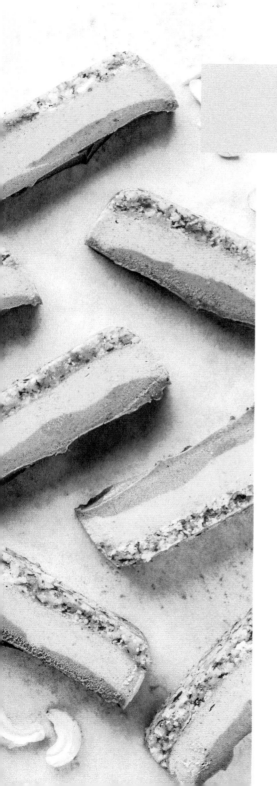

CONTENTS

CONTENTS

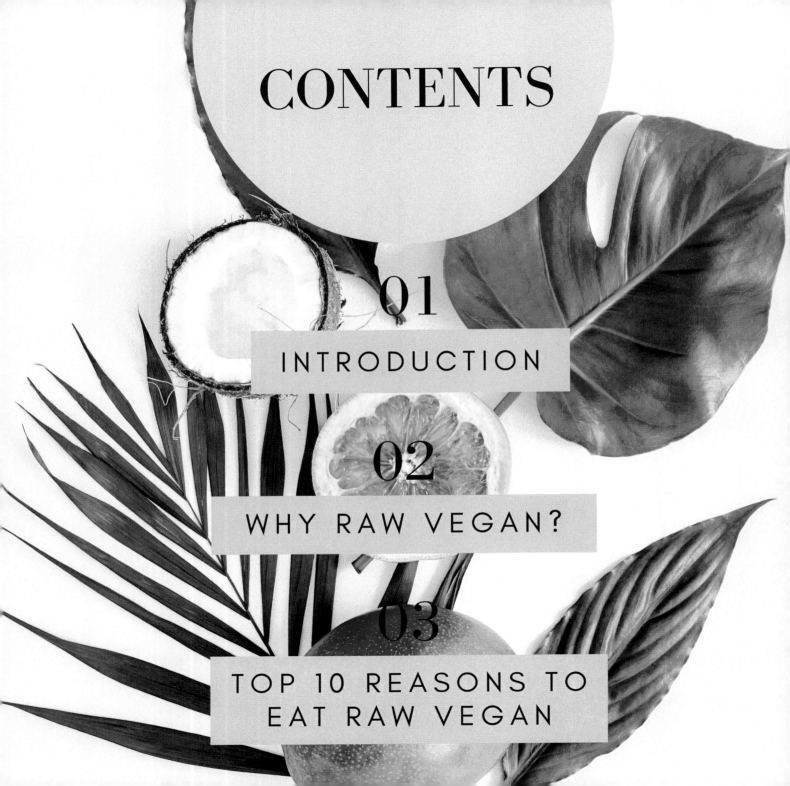

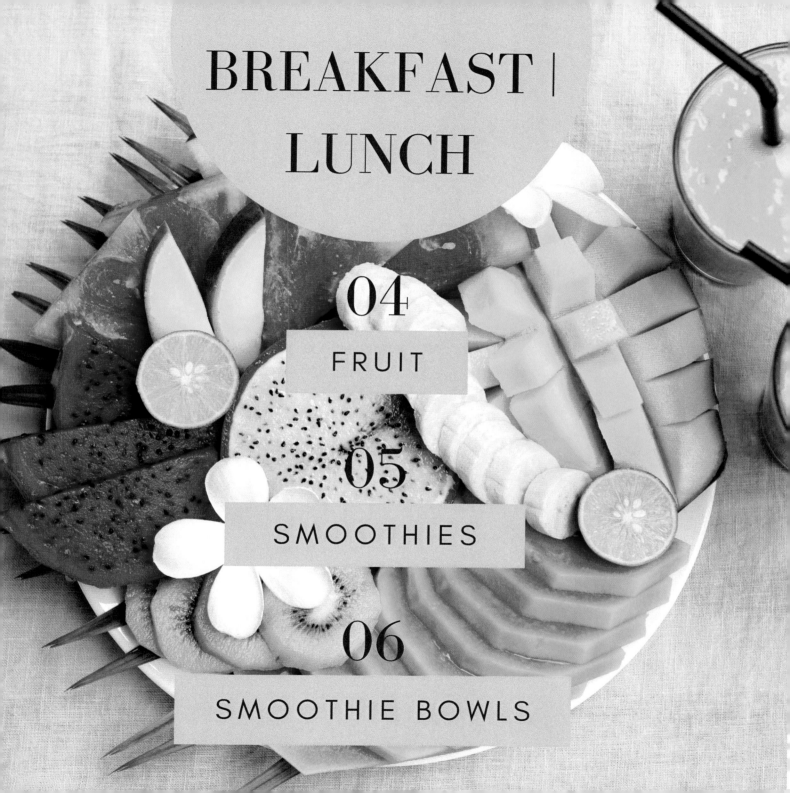

BREAKFAST | LUNCH

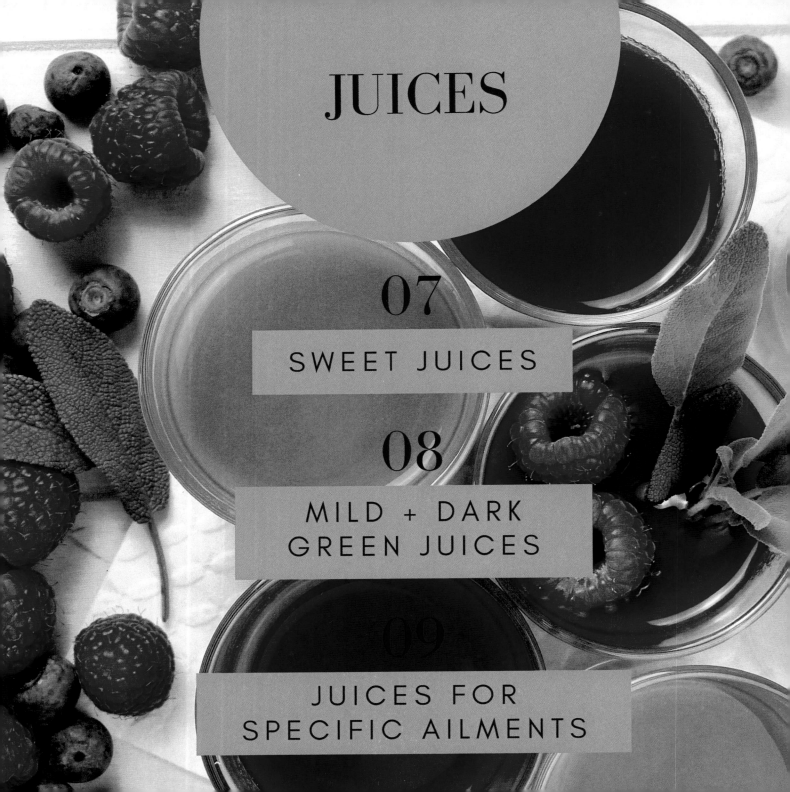

JUICES

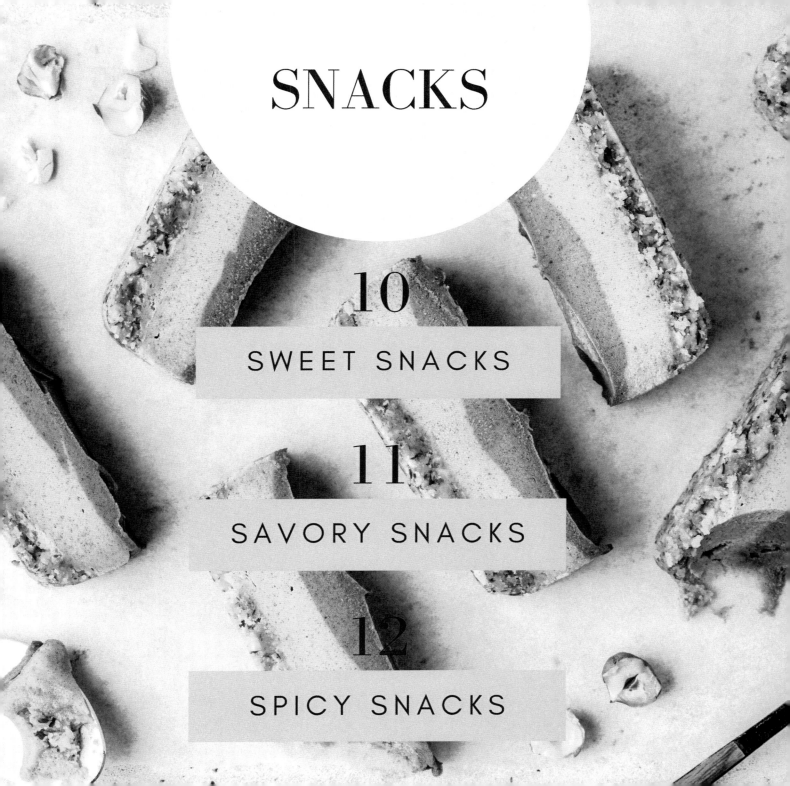

SNACKS

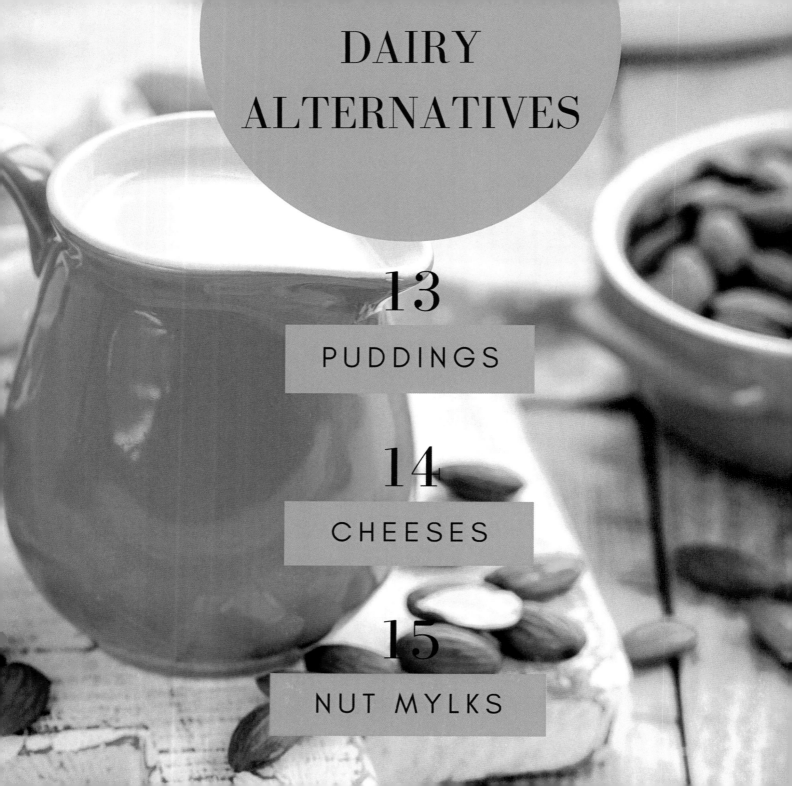

DAIRY ALTERNATIVES

DINNER

16

ENTREES | WRAPS
PASTA | SUSHI+

17

SALAD DRESSINGS

18

DIPS

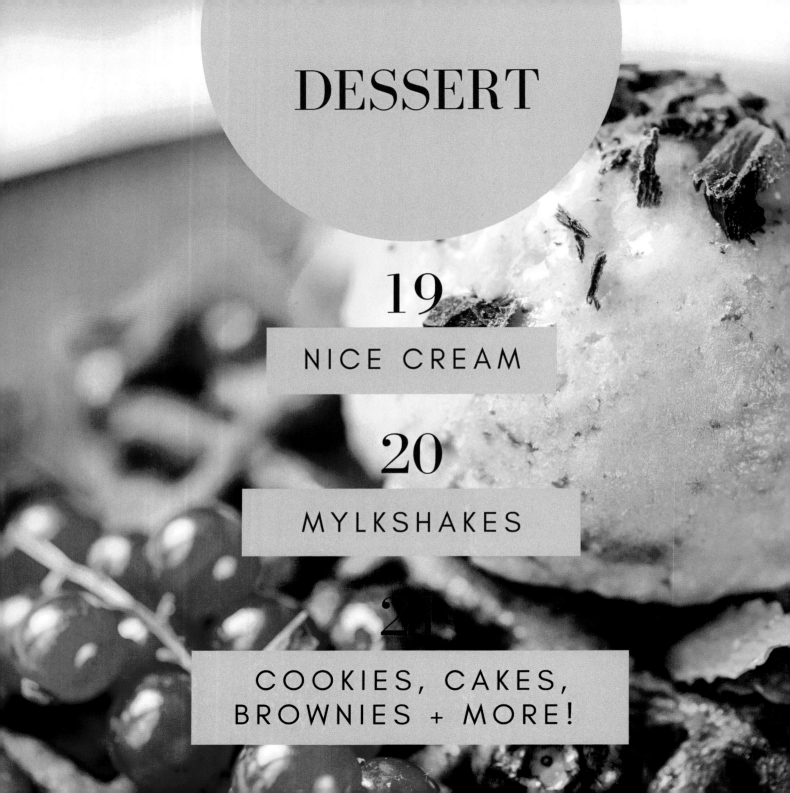

DESSERT

19
NICE CREAM

20
MYLKSHAKES

21
COOKIES, CAKES, BROWNIES + MORE!

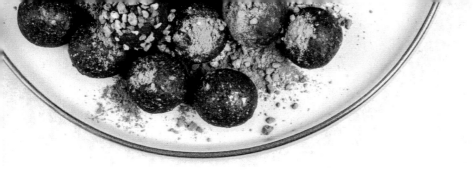

INTRODUCTION

Being healthy and eating a raw vegan diet does not have to be complicated!

I organized this book as a resource containing all of my favorite recipes created over the past 13 years while living a raw vegan lifestyle. I felt called to do this especially because most of the raw food books that I have read contain complicated recipes with lots of ingredients and require excessive time in the kitchen and/or a dehydrator.

Honestly, I do own a dehydrator but I've used it only a handful of times since going raw in 2011. Personally, I do not enjoy spending hours upon hours constructing raw vegan food in the kitchen. Recipes that seem to never end and take 18+ hours to dehydrate are not my thing! I enjoy it most and feel my best eating simple and delicious food. This is the reason most of these recipes came to fruition. Some even have only 2 ingredients!

Thank you for taking the time to check out this book. I hope you make some of these recipes and love them as much as I do!

If you'd like, feel free to tag me on any recipes you make!
I'd LOVE to see your gorgeous creations!

Jeannette | @Ms.FitVegan

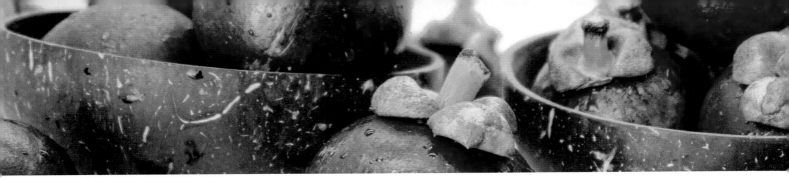

WHY RAW?

In order to feel energetic, healthy, vibrant and alive... we need to eat as much raw food as possible!

The reason is simple:

We Are What We Eat!

If we consume mostly cooked and processed (dead food)... we will feel mostly cooked and dead. If we eat an abundance of food that is alive with vitamins, minerals, and nutrients... we will feel alive and full of energy!

When food is cooked above 118 degrees, the food loses most of its vitamins and minerals. Cooking destroys the live enzymes and life force of food. This then doesn't allow us to get the benefits from the food we eat!

When we eat the best foods on earth (raw, fresh, ripe fruit and veggies) we feel the best we've EVER felt!

Eating a diet consisting of fruit, vegetables, nuts, and seeds while eliminating meat, dairy, grains, and processed food allows us to not only be in the best health of our life, but it also helps us naturally heal any ailments we may be currently suffering from.

Our digestive system consumes approximately 70% of our total energy. Eating a diet of fresh, raw, uncooked, unprocessed food that is easy to digest - allows for our bodies to focus on healing whatever needs attention, instead of consistently expending most of its energy digesting the unhealthy food we've consumed.

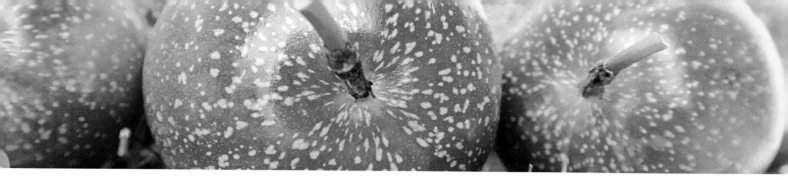

WHY RAW?

TOP 10 REASONS TO TRY A RAW VEGAN DIET FOR ONE WEEK

MOOD

Are you someone who has mood swings? Do you wake up some days super depressed and other days excited and happy? Do little things get to you? Do you find yourself being mean and disrespectful to the people that you love the most? This may sound crazy but a raw vegan diet can help you be in a better, happier and more stable mood! You are what you eat right? So if you are eating things with zero live enzymes, zero life force, zero nutrition, fried in oil, or (God forbid) you are eating dead animal body parts... the emotions and energy that were in the animal (right before it was killed) are still in its muscle tissues. Energy can never die, it can only be transferred. When you eat things with fear in it, you absorb that fear. When you eat junk food, you will feel like junk. When you eat heavy fatty foods, you will feel heavy and fat. Even skinny people that look healthy on the outside, do not feel good, happy or healthy after they eat junk food. There is a price for everything, always! Remember this!

On the opposite side of the spectrum, when you eat foods with vibrant colors, rich in vitamins, minerals and nutrients, foods that are alive with the sun's energy (all fruit and vegetables contain energy from the sun) then you will FEEL that loving, calm, peaceful energy that they contain. Studies have proven there is a direct correlation between food, mood, and violent behavior. There is also a direct correlation between food and depression. But don't take my word for it. Try eating raw vegan for one week and see for yourself!

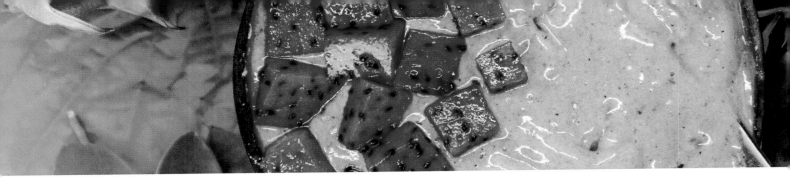

WHY RAW?

ENERGY

Put the best in to get the best out! Would you buy a Rolls Royce and put the cheapest fuel in? No way! So why in the world do we put crap into our bodies and expect it to perform at a high level? Are our bodies not WAY more valuable and MORE important than a car? Would you rather lose all your extremities or have the car of your dreams? Perspective is humbling isn't it?

Are there things in life that you want to have or accomplish but you have no idea how you are going to muster up the energy to make these things happen? There is literally NO OTHER LIFESTYLE on the planet that will give you as much energy as a raw vegan diet! Now I'm not saying you are banned from ever eating cooked food. After trying raw for one week, if you want to go back to cooked food you absolutely can. A 100% raw vegan lifestyle is not for everyone, so if you don't LOVE how it feels and how your food tastes then go back to eating some healthy cooked food, by all means. But there is no reason you can't experience the amazing benefits of eating MOSTLY raw! Arnold Ehret in his revolutionary book "The Mucusless Diet Healing System" stated that a diet containing 51% raw and 49% cooked is better than 51% cooked and 49% raw. Very wise! That 2% difference can be a GAME CHANGER for you! Try eating raw vegan for one week, after that - if you miss cooked food, then consider eating a raw vegan breakfast and lunch and then having some healthy cooked fruit or vegetables in a huge salad with a delicious dressing for dinner. Try this out. This is called Raw Till 4. In my humble opinion, this is the second most healthiest lifestyle on the planet, right behind the raw vegan diet. Raw till 4 is also extremely socially acceptable and doable. If you are a very social person, it may be weird and inconvenient to always be bringing fruit or raw food to parties, restaurants, etc. This is what I do but I totally understand that is not for everyone!

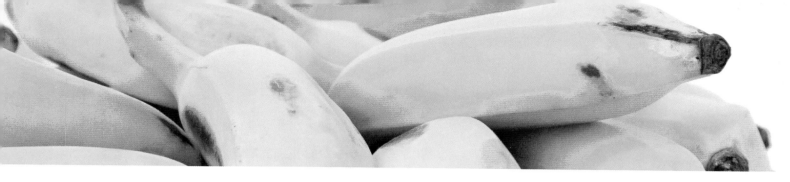

WHY RAW?

CLEAR BEAUTIFUL SKIN

What is going on inside your body shows on the outside! And what your skin looks like is a direct result of the state of your colon. There are no if, ands, or butts, about it. Pun intended.

Oily skin? You're eating to much oils and high fatty foods. Dry skin? You are dehydrated and eating a lot of low water content foods like bread, crackers, meat, etc. Do you suffer with acne? Have you always dreamed of having beautiful skin and not having to wear foundation or concealer? Do you wish you could just be blessed with naturally clear glowing skin? I'm here to share that you can have it but you have to work for it. Just like everything in life. **Everything works IF you do the work!**

Clear skin was my number one goal when I started eating raw vegan. I wanted to lose weight, I wanted to stop feeling depressed, I wanted more energy, but I NEEDED to clear my skin. My struggle with acne began at the age of 12, and it became a significant source of anxiety an embarrassment for me! Even with pounds of makeup on my face, I was still so embarrassed, ashamed and self-conscious that I missed many days of school and was almost kicked out of Junior High School. I tried everything - every cream, prescription pill, face mask, everything! Absolutely nothing worked until I was 26 years old and I discovered the Raw Vegan Lifestyle. Raw Foods completed healed my cystic acne that I suffered with for over 10 years of my life and it has never returned! You do not have to suffer. Please consider a raw food diet and watch your skin become clear, glowing and the skin you always dreamed of having!

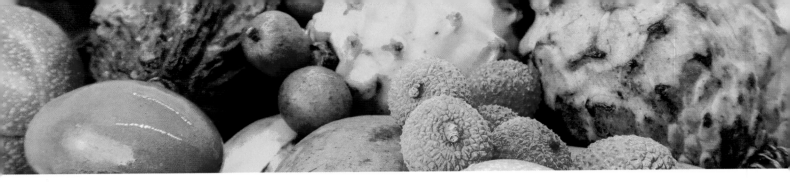

WHY RAW?

SLEEP

If you sleep a lot it probably means you are eating a lot of crap. Aside from depression, being tired and needing a lot of sleep is usually a sign that your body is busy trying to digest all the crap you put inside of it during the day. Now, as a raw vegan for over 14 years... I TRY to sleep for 8 hours...and I can not. No alarm clock needed! My body just does not want to oversleep. If you want to get up fully energized every morning and not wake up tired, try the raw vegan lifestyle! Especially if you are going from a meat and junk food diet to a raw vegan diet... your entire life will change!

FOCUS

No more cloudiness or brain fog for your fruity cutie! I have never EVER been as sharp as I am now! I WISH I was raw vegan when I was in school! If you are in school, start eating more fresh fruit and vegetables, it will be an automatic game changer for you!!!!! Our brains run exclusively on glucose. The cleanest, most efficient source of glucose is fructose. The healthiest source of fructose is, yes you guessed it, fruit

BATHROOM ISSUES BE GONE!

If you have stomach or bathroom issues... increase the amount of fruit and veggies you eat and start to eliminate everything else! If you are constipated - you are dehydrated! Water isn't really hydration. H2O water is dead. However, the H3O inside of fruit and vegetables is living electrolytes with real powerful hydration. After just one week of eating a raw vegan diet you will see your bathroom situation improve drastically. Imagine if you went raw vegan for a month or an entire year? And if you don't think you have any bathroom issues... does it smell really bad after you go? That is very bad sign of what is going on in your body! Poop is NOT supposed to smell bad!

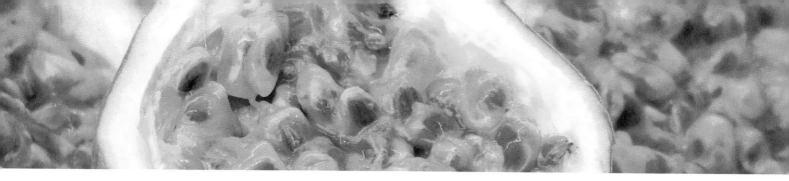

WHY RAW?

BAD BREATH | BODY ODOR

What is going on inside your body comes out on the outside. The digestive system is simply just one long tube from our mouth to our anus. If your breath smells, you have rotting and putrefying old decaying fecal matter inside of you. If you are consuming animal products though, bad breath is the least of your problems to be honest. Animal products are scientifically proven to be the LEADING cause of all preventable diseases including cancer, heart disease, strokes, diabetes, and more. **What goes up must come down but what goes into your body doesn't always come out.** Eating raw vegan will help to liquefy the old decaying fecal matter inside your large and small intestines and allow it to be released. This old toxic decaying matter is the cause of your stinky bowels, bad breath, smelly farts and body odor! We live one life. The way I see it - while 'm here, I don't want to have bad breath, stink or deal with nasty odors coming from my body. Put the best in - get the best out!

As my fruity cuties say... Eat Fruit and Be Cute!!! :)

WEIGHT LOSS CATALYST | MARK THE BEGINNING OF A HEALTHIER YOU | A HEALTHIER LIFESTYLE

There is no better lifestyle on earth for losing weight than the raw vegan diet. It is the only lifestyle I've ever been able to stick with long enough to see weight loss! Here is why... this lifestyle is one where you can eat as much as you want as long as your food is made from fruit, vegetables, nuts, seeds, spices, herbs or seaweed. Fruit is extremely sweet and the healthier you become, the more sweet it tastes, and the more you crave it! Our taste buds change every seven days, so all you have to do is eat and abundance of fruit and veggies for seven days to start craving more of them! **Whatever is in our blood stream is what we will crave!** One of the biggest tips I can give you is to stop consuming something if you want to stop craving it!

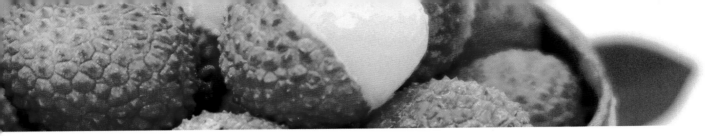

WHY RAW?

STRENGTHENS YOUR IMMUNE SYSTEM!

Choosing to eat raw is the fastest way to healing ANYTHING – from a paper cut to cancer. While eating raw vegan you will notice your ENTIRE body healing so much quicker than EVER before! Healing quickly is a sign that your immune system is strong. I have not needed to take antibiotics in over 14 years.. and I never ever get sick. Every year people round me get sick and I somehow never catch it... why? Because my immune system is strong. Even the most extremely contagious diseases cannot be contracted if your immune system is strong!

RAW GIVES YOU MORE TIME & MAKES YOUR LIFE EASIER!

I started saving so much time not cooking! The time you spend cooking could be spent learning new things, playing with family, or doing things you love and making a difference in this world! I know it may not seem like you are spending a lot of time in the kitchen but trust me you will notice the HUGE amount of free time you save by not cooking! Its true that gourmet raw food takes a hell of a lot of time but eating meals of fruit and veggies in their natural state is so ridiculously easy. And that is exactly how I do it! Sometime I do smoothies and they take less than 5 minutes.

Raw makes your life EASIER because being overweight sick and unhealthy is really really hard! Eating raw makes your body, mind and spirit lighter and feel better so that you can live the life you were meant to live! I have been on both sides now and I promise you – life is way EASIER raw!

In life, you can have excuses or results my friend. But you can NEVER have both!

My goal in creating this book is to help you NEVER make another excuse again. With these simple, easy and delicious recipes you can easily be healthy, look glowing and gorgeous and feel AMAZING every single day for the rest of your life! So let's begin!

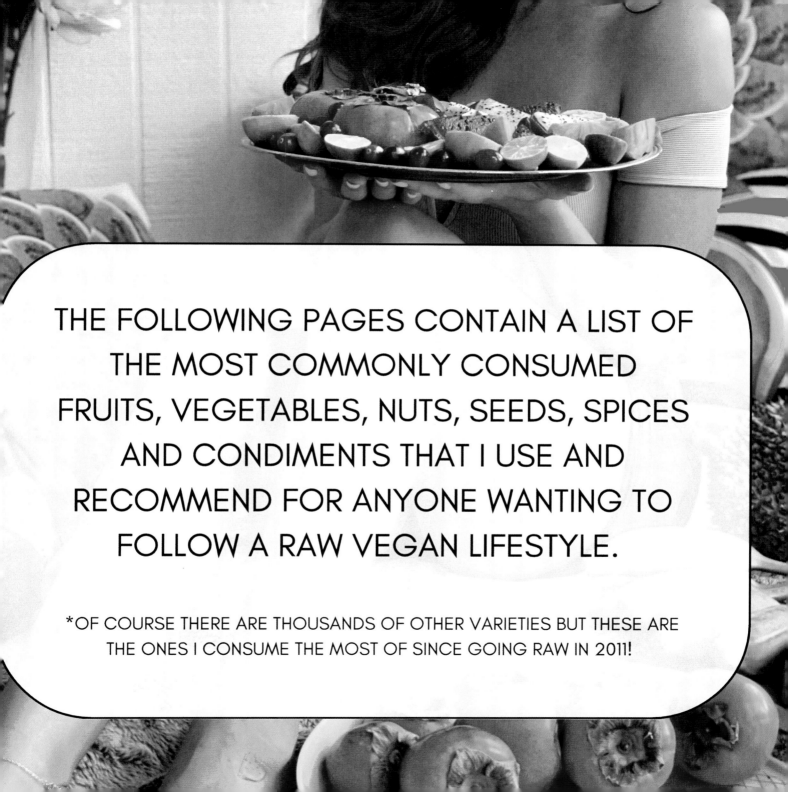

THE FOLLOWING PAGES CONTAIN A LIST OF THE MOST COMMONLY CONSUMED FRUITS, VEGETABLES, NUTS, SEEDS, SPICES AND CONDIMENTS THAT I USE AND RECOMMEND FOR ANYONE WANTING TO FOLLOW A RAW VEGAN LIFESTYLE.

*OF COURSE THERE ARE THOUSANDS OF OTHER VARIETIES BUT THESE ARE THE ONES I CONSUME THE MOST OF SINCE GOING RAW IN 2011!

FRUITS

- Acai
- Ackee
- Apples
- Apricots
- Avocados
- Baby Bananas
- Bananas
- Bell Peppers
- Blackberry
- Blackcurrant
- Blueberries
- Boysenberry
- Breadfruit
- Cactus Fruit
- Cantaloupe
- Chayote
- Cherimoya
- Cherries
- Clementine
- Coconut
- Cranberries
- Cucumbers
- Currants
- Dates
- Dragon Fruit (Pitaya)
- Durian
- Elderberry
- Feijoa
- Figs
- Gooseberry
- Grapes
- Grapefruit
- Guava
- Honeydew
- Jackfruit
- Jabuticaba

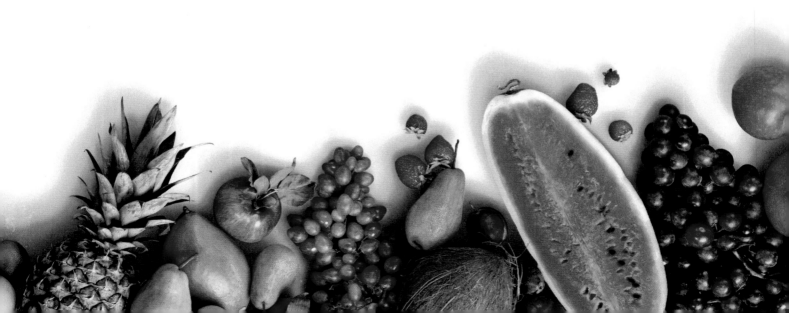

FRUITS

- Kiwis
- Kumquat
- Langsat
- Lemons
- Limes
- Longans
- Lychee
- Mamey Sapote
- Mamoncillo
- Mangoes
- Mangosteen
- Melons (all varieties)
- Mulberry
- Nectarines
- Oranges
- Papaya
- Passion Fruit
- Peaches
- Pears
- Persimmons
- Pineapple
- Plum
- Pomegranate
- Pomelo
- Rambutan
- Raspberries
- Red Currants
- Santol
- Sapodilla
- Soursop
- Star Fruit
- Strawberry
- Tamarind
- Tangerines
- Tomatoes
- Ugli Fruit
- Watermelon
- Zucchinis

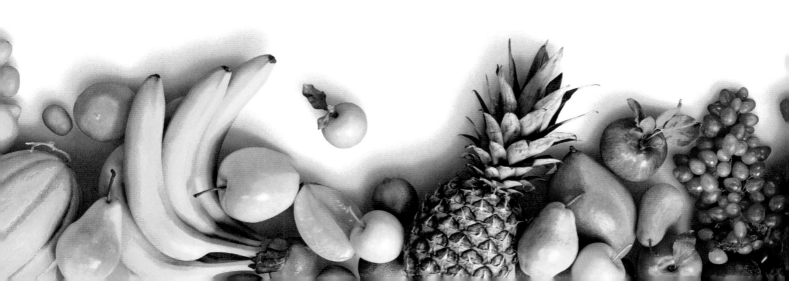

GREEN LEAFY VEGETABLES

- Arugula (Rocket)
- Baby Kale
- Baby Spinach
- Beet Greens
- Butterhead Lettuce (includes Boston and Bibb varieties)
- Cabbage (Green)
- Collard Greens
- Dandelion Greens
- Endive
- Escarole
- Fiddlehead Ferns
- Green Leaf Lettuce
- Iceberg Lettuce
- Kale
- Microgreens
- Mizuna
- Mustard Greens
- Mustard Spinach (Komatsuna)
- Napa Cabbage
- Radicchio
- Red Leaf Lettuce
- Romaine Lettuce
- Savoy Cabbage
- Sorrel
- Spinach
- Swiss Chard
- Tatsoi
- Turnip Greens
- Watercress

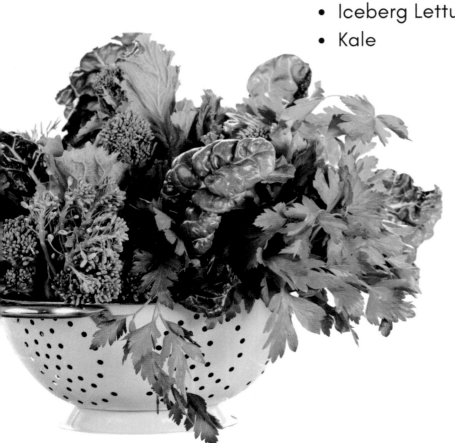

VEGETABLES

- Artichoke
- Arugula (Rocket)
- Asparagus
- Beets (Beetroot)
- Bok Choy (Pak Choi)
- Broccoli
- Broccoli Rabe (Rapini)
- Brussels Sprouts
- Cabbage (Green, Red, Savoy)
- Carrots
- Cauliflower
- Celery
- Chicory
- Corn (Maize)
- Daikon Radish
- Eggplant (Aubergine)
- Endive
- Fennel
- Garlic
- Green Beans
- Jicama
- Kohlrabi
- Leeks
- Mushrooms
- Okra
- Onions (Red, White, Yellow)
- Parsnips
- Peas
- Pumpkin
- Radishes
- Rhubarb
- Rutabaga
- Scallions (Green Onions)
- Shallots
- Turnips

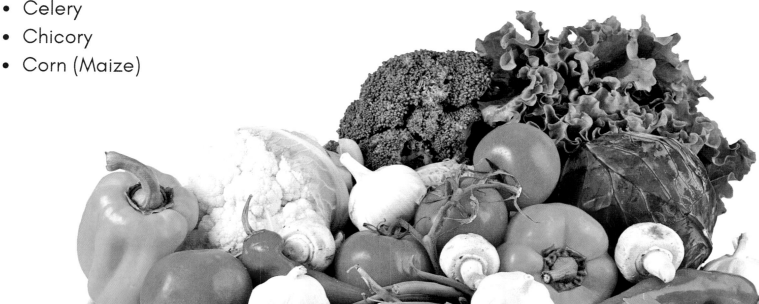

RECOMMENDED STORE-BOUGHT CONDIMENTS

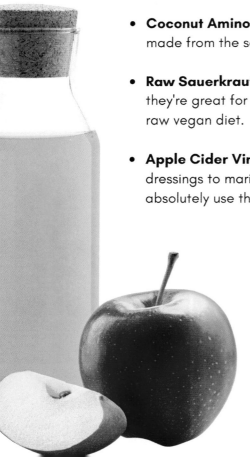

- **Nutritional Yeast:** It's a popular cheese substitute in the raw vegan world due to its savory, cheesy flavor. Please be sure to only use a non-fortified brand as like LOOV Organic, Sari Foods, Foods Alive, etc. Fortified nutritional yeast contains synthetic vitamins which are made in a science lab! No thanks!

- **Nama Shoyu:** This is a raw, unpasteurized soy sauce. It is often used in raw vegan recipes for an umami flavor.

- **Coconut Aminos:** A salty, slightly sweet sauce that's often used as a soy sauce substitute. It's made from the sap of coconut palms. The sap is fermented and then blended with sea salt.

- **Raw Sauerkraut or Kimchi:** Fermented foods like these can be a tasty addition to a meal, and they're great for gut health. Make sure to look for raw and unpasteurized versions to fit within a raw vegan diet.

- **Apple Cider Vinegar:** A versatile ingredient that can be used in many recipes, from salad dressings to marinades. I prefer to use lemon or lime as a ACV replacement but you can absolutely use this if desired.

- **Mustard:** While many commercially available mustards are not raw, there are a few brands that sell raw mustard. You can also simply use mustard seeds instead of mustard. I only use the mustards with real ingredients, no chemicals, citric acid or preservatives.

- **Nut and Seed Butters:** Such as almond butter, cashew butter, tahini, or sunflower seed butter. Look for brands that are raw and don't contain any added oils or sugars. I get my nuts, seeds and nut butters from ww.LivingNutz.com

SWEETENERS

Here are 5 sweeteners I recommend. However, fresh fruit is the absolute best and healthiest option!

- **Fresh Fruit:** Bananas, Pineapple, Apples, Pears, etc. Really any sweet fruit will make an excellent sweetener for any recipe!

- **Dried Fruit:** Dates, dried figs, raisins, dried apricots or dried mulberries make excellent sweeteners. Soak for at least 20 minutes if you need them to be soft to blend easier in recipes!

- **Date Syrup:** You can buy this in most grocery stores however I'd recommend you make your own. Simply blend equal parts dates and water. You can also freeze this liquid into an ice cube tray and use a date cubes whenever you need a sweetener. I recommend FRESH dates from bautistaorganicdates.com because most of the dates in the stores are old, dry and rancid!

- **Stevia:** Stevia is a natural sweetener derived from the leaves of the Stevia rebaudiana plant, which is native to South America, specifically Paraguay and Brazil. The plant has been used for centuries by indigenous people to sweeten food and beverages. Stevia is natural but I do not like the after taste so I do not use it! If you lie it then this may be a good option for you!

- **Monk Fruit:** Monk fruit sweetener is made by extracting the juice from the monk fruit (also known as luo han guo). The purified extract is often dried into a powder form, sometimes mixed with other ingredients like erythritol or dextrose to balance the sweetness and improve texture for use in recipes.

SWEETENERS I WOULD NOT RECOMMEND USING

These sweeteners are processed and contain NO FIBER, therefor unnaturally spiking your blood sugar, giving you cravings and making you MORE hungry!

- **Maple Syrup:** Make sure it is organic and 100% pure Grade A maple syrup. I prefer to use fruit as sweetener but feel free to use maple syrup if you absolutely must. Maple syrup is made by collecting sap from sugar maple trees and boiling it down to concentrate the natural sugars into a thick, flavorful syrup. THERE IS NO SUCH THING AS RAW MAPLE SYRUP!

- **Agave:** Agave syrup is highly processed through enzymatic and heat treatments to convert its natural starches and inulin into concentrated fructose. **THERE IS NO SUCH THING AS RAW AGAVE** and this sweetener should be avoided at all cost.

- **Cane Sugar:** Cane sugar is processed by crushing sugarcane, extracting the juice, and refining it through multiple stages of heating, filtering, and crystallizing to produce pure sucrose.

- **Brown Sugar:** Brown sugar is made by mixing white sugar with molasses or by leaving some molasses in the sugar during the refining process.

- **Molasses:** Molasses is a byproduct of refining sugarcane or sugar beets, involving boiling and extracting sugar crystals, which strips away natural fiber and concentrates the sugar.

SEAWEED

Here is a list of popular seaweeds that can be a helpful addition in the raw vegan diet when you are craving salt!

- **Nori:** This seaweed is often used in sushi rolls and snacks. It's high in vitamins A and C.

- **Kombu:** Used in a variety of dishes, especially soups and stews. Kombu is often used to make dashi, a Japanese broth.

- **Wakame:** Frequently used in miso soup and salads. It's a good source of iodine, calcium, and vitamins A, C, E, and K.

- **Dulse (my fav):** This red seaweed is often used in soups, salads, and sandwiches. It's high in protein, fiber, and vitamins.

- **Arame:** Typically used in salads and stir-fries. It's a great source of calcium, iodine, iron, magnesium, and vitamin A.

- **Hijiki:** This seaweed is often used in salads, stir-fries, and soups. It's a good source of dietary fiber and essential minerals.

- **Irish Sea Moss:** This seaweed is often used as a thickening agent in vegan dishes and is a source of various minerals.

- **Sea Lettuce:** As the name suggests, this green seaweed can be used in salads and soups.

- **Agar:** It's derived from red algae and is often used as a gelatin substitute in vegan cooking.

- **Spirulina:** Often sold in powdered form, it's a nutrient-dense superfood that can be added to smoothies.

RECOMMENDED HOMEMADE CONDIMENTS

*Please note that all of these condiment recipes are found in this book!

- **Guacamole:** Made from avocados, lime juice, and various seasonings. You can add ingredients like fresh tomatoes, red onions, cilantro, and jalapeno peppers for added flavor.

- **Salsa:** tomatoes, onions, chilies, cilantro, and lime juice.

- **Pesto:** Made from fresh basil, parsley, pine nuts or walnuts, garlic, lemon juice and water.

- **Tomato Sauces:** Such as marinara sauce made from sundried and fresh tomatoes, dates, and fresh herbs.

- **Hummus:** zucchini, lemon, garlic, hemp or pumpkin seeds, green onion, and sun dried tomatoes

- **Fruit Purees:** These can be used as spreads or sweeteners and can be made from any fruit you like + dates.

- **Salad Dressings:** Made with nuts, seeds, fruits, vegetables, lemon or lime juice, and herbs and spices.

- **Raw Vegan Mayo:** Made from raw cashews or macadamia nuts, lemon juice, a bit of sweetener like dates or maple syrup.

- **Raw Vegan Cheese:** Made from nuts or seeds like cashews or sunflower seeds, nutritional yeast, and various seasonings.

SPICES

Many spices can be used in a raw vegan diet to enhance the flavor of dishes. Here's a list of some of my most used spices:

- **Basil:** Fresh basil leaves are great in salads, pestos, and other dishes.

- **Black Pepper:** Used in a variety of dishes to enhance flavor.

- **Cardamom:** Great in both sweet and savory dishes.

- **Cayenne Pepper:** Adds a bit of heat to dishes.

- **Cinnamon:** Often used in sweet dishes or smoothies.

- **Cloves:** Often used in desserts, but also good in savory dishes.

- **Coriander:** Used in both its seed form and as fresh cilantro leaves.

- **Cumin:** Adds an earthy flavor to many dishes.

- **Dill:** Fresh or dried, it's often used in raw vegan dips and sauces.

- **Ginger:** Can be used fresh or dried and adds a zesty kick to dishes.

- **Mint:** Fresh leaves can add a cool, refreshing note to salads, smoothies, or desserts.

- **Nutmeg:** Commonly used in desserts or sprinkled on top of sweet dishes.

- **Pink Himalayan Salt:** Preferred by many raw vegans over regular table salt due to its mineral content. Use this sparingly and only if necessary.

- **Smoked paprika:** Not technically raw but adds such a delicious flavor to salad dressings!

- **Turmeric:** Known for its anti-inflammatory properties, it's often used in juices or dressings.

- **Vanilla:** Vanilla beans, paste, or raw vanilla powder can add a sweet, floral flavor to desserts.

NUTS & SEEDS

Try your very best to always consume nuts and seeds raw, un roasted, and without salt!

- Almonds
- Beech nuts
- Brazil nuts
- Butternuts
- Cashews
- Chestnuts
- Hazelnuts
- Litchi nuts
- Macadamia nuts
- Peanuts
- Pecans
- Pine nuts
- Pistachios
- Walnuts

- Chia seeds
- Flaxseeds
- Hemp seeds
- Pumpkin seeds
- Sunflower seeds
- Sesame seeds

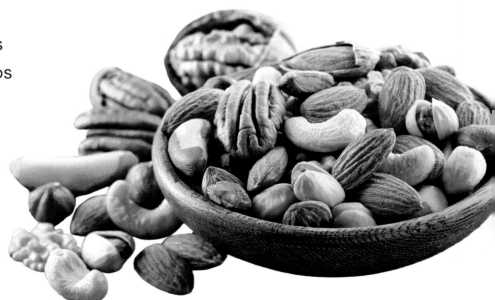

WHY WE DON'T WANT TO CONSUME SALT

Always use salt sparingly and only if and when necessary.

Here are 10 lesser-known reasons to avoid salt, specifically for raw vegans who already have a solid foundation in nutrition:

1. Cellular Dehydration: Salt pulls water out of cells to balance extracellular sodium levels, leaving cells dehydrated. This cellular dehydration can affect energy production and enzyme activity, impacting overall cellular health.

2. Interferes with Electrolyte Balance: Excess salt can disrupt the body's natural electrolyte balance, which may interfere with nerve function and muscle contractions—key concerns for those consuming high-water-content fruits and veggies.

3. Inhibits Stomach Acid Production: High salt intake can inhibit the body's ability to produce hydrochloric acid in the stomach, affecting digestion and nutrient absorption, especially critical for raw vegans reliant on efficient digestion.

4. Contributes to Microbiome Imbalance: Salt can negatively impact gut microbiota diversity by reducing certain beneficial bacteria, potentially affecting immune health and mood due to the gut-brain connection.

WHY WE DON'T WANT TO CONSUME SALT

6. Leaches Potassium from the Body: High sodium intake can force the body to lose potassium, which is essential for muscle function, heart health, and preventing fatigue—an imbalance particularly impactful for raw vegans who prioritize natural potassium sources.

7. Stimulates Adrenal Glands: Salt consumption can lead to overstimulation of the adrenal glands, causing stress on the endocrine system and potentially leading to adrenal fatigue, especially in those already committed to a lower-stress, natural lifestyle.

8. Impairs Cognitive Function: Excess salt can increase oxidative stress in the brain, potentially impairing memory and cognitive function over time—a lesser-known connection between sodium and brain health.

9. May Increase Risk of Stomach Cancer: Salt irritates the stomach lining, creating a hostile environment that could promote stomach cancer. This risk persists even with natural salts, as it's the sodium content itself that's irritating.

10. Reduces Natural Hydration Signals: Salt consumption can dull the body's natural thirst signals, leading people to drink less water than their body actually needs, counteracting the natural hydration focus of a raw diet. Instead of salt... drink green juice, eat more greens and add seasweed to your diet! It will help with the salty cravings!

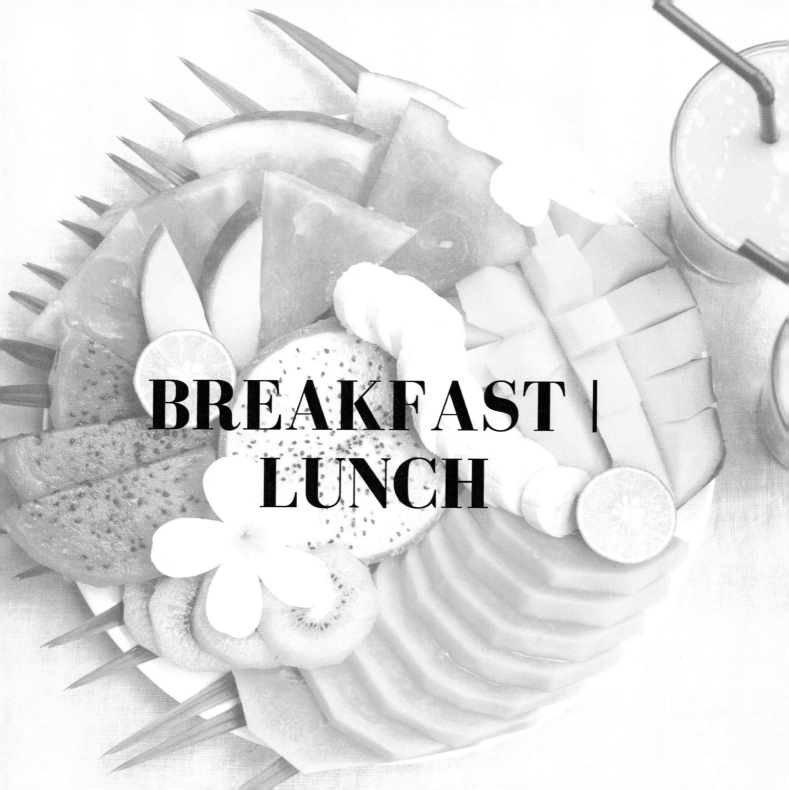

BREAKFAST | LUNCH

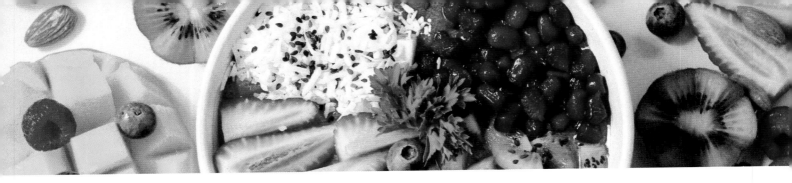

BREAKFAST

MONO MEAL - A MEAL COMPRISED SOLELY OF ONE FOOD, PREFERABLY RAW FRUITS

Fruit is THE BEST and most optimal food to eat for breakfast! Specifically, I want to encourage you to eat a mono-meal of your favorite in-season fruit as the first thing you eat each day. There are so many benefits to eating mono-meals!

Different enzymes are needed to break down different food types including proteins, carbohydrates, fats and sugars. If too much activity is happening in the digestive tract, acids can counteract the enzymes, causing food to ferment as opposed to being digested.

And with so many different ingredients consumed in one sitting, it can be a tiring process for our bodies to complete. Some side effects of eating too many ingredients at once include heartburn, lethargy and gastrointestinal disturbances. Have you ever ate watermelon until you were full? If so, you've eaten a mono meal. Your body will receive this food in oneness and in wholeness, causing it to trigger one enzymatic reaction to successfully digest it!

Benefits of Eating a Mono-Meal of Fruit For Breakfast:

1. Better digestion!
2. Less bloating!
3. Less gas!
4. More satisfied!
5. Less chance that you will overeat (when you eat a mono meal your body stops when its full and doesn't go beyond that point!)
6. More energy throughout the day!
7. Clearer skin!
8. No recipe is required!
9. Easy and saves you time!
10. Eliminates decision fatigue!
11. Allows you to enjoy the simplicity of just one food--the taste, texture, smell, etc! (the way nature intended)
12. Makes it easy to eat healthy on the go!
13. Re-trains your taste buds to enjoy natural, healthy sugar!
14. Re-trains your brain to know when you're full!
15. Can be applied for an extended period of time as a detox or cleanse!
16. Helps to retrain your grelin and leptin receptors!

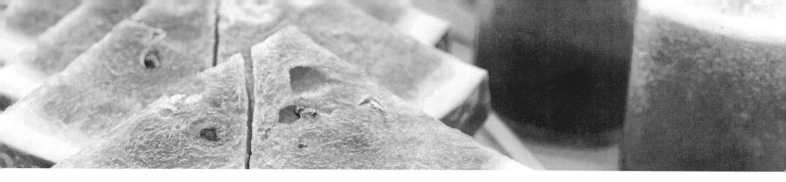

FRUIT

Best Mono-Meal Breakfast Ideas:

Watermelon

Any other type of melon

Persimmons

(must be extremely ripe)

Papaya

Mangoes

Longans

Rambutan

Lychees

Oranges

Apples

Grapes

Pineapple

(must be extremely ripe)

Figs

(must be extremely ripe)

White or Red Dragon Fruit

Soursop

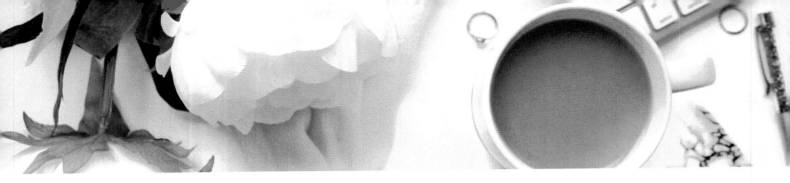

COFFEE REPLACEMENT

Caffeine is one of the most dangerous and addicting substances in the world. It should be illegal. It destroys our adrenal glands, thyroid functions, metabolism, digestive system, nervous system, and more! As a healthy alternative, I recommend the following all-natural coffee replacement:

Hot Date Latte

Ingredients

6 medjool dates
Fresh ginger juice or a small piece of
fresh ginger
1/2 tsp cinnamon
10oz hot water

Directions

1. De-pit the dates and place into the blender
2. Add ginger, dates, and cinnamon to the blender
3. Heat water until it is boiling hot and add to blender
4. Blend until frothy
5. Pour and top with a few sprinkles of cinnamon

Tips and tricks:

*Experiment! Use more dates to make it creamier and less for a thinner consistency. Add more ginger or cinnamon to taste!

*Heat your favorite nut milk and use it instead of water for an even creamier consistency.

*Add maca, spirulina, Daily Green Boost, your favorite green powder, or any energizing supplements for an even added boost of energy when drinking.

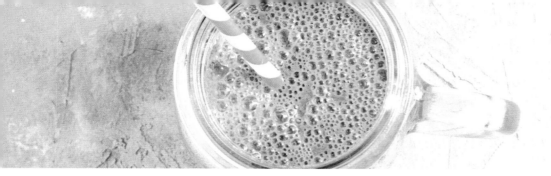

SMOOTHIES

All recipes are designed to create 32oz smoothies. I recommend to double the food recipe (and add more liquid to blender as desired) if you are having these as meals. Yes you read that right! A 64oz smoothie is a meal. Not a 32oz smoothie! However, feel free to use the exact 32oz recipe if you are having smoothies as a snack or you're not very hungry!

Please note that all liquid bases can be substituted for the base of your choice. You can use ANY type of plant based mylk, coconut water and/or simply just plain filter or distilled or spring water. You can even do 1/2 nut mylk and 1/2 water to make it a lighter smoothie if you'd like! Substituting water for nut mylk will change the consistency of the smoothie.

My favorite nut mylks to use are: hemp, coconut, almond, walnut, and cashew. You can purchase nut mylk in the store (make sure it is Carrageenan free!) or you can make your own! I often ad a TBSP of hemp seeds directly to my smoothie, add water and it comes out delicious and creamy!

Equipment you will need:

High-Speed Powered Blender
Very Thin Strainer or a Nut Mylk Bag
Wisk or Spatula
Large Bottle with Lid (Preferably glass as nut mylk will last longer!)

Nut Mylk Recipe

1 cup of any nut of your choice (or 3 TBSP of any nut butter of your choice!)
3 cups water
1-2 dates (optional)
1" vanilla bean (optional)

See the Dairy Alternatives section for my almond mylk recipe!

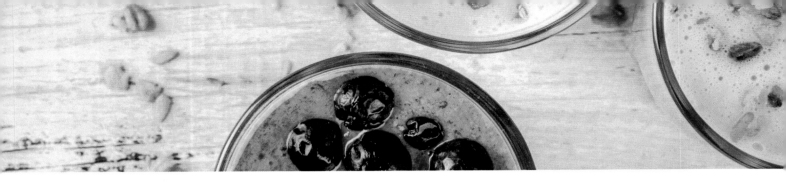

SMOOTHIES

The Energizing Blend

A delicious and creamy tropical green smoothie

24 oz water or any nut mylk of your choice
1 cup of spinach or kale
5 frozen bananas
1 cup frozen mango
1/2 cup frozen pineapple

The Invigorating Blend

A green smoothie that tastes like mint chip ice cream

1 drop peppermint spirits or peppermint oil (put in first)
24 oz water or any nut mylk of your choice
5 frozen bananas
1 cup spinach or kale
2 tbsp caco nibs
Add in 2 medjool dates if you'd like it extra sweet!

Place cacao nibs in blender **after** blending and everything is smooth! Blend with cacao nibs for 5-10 seconds only!

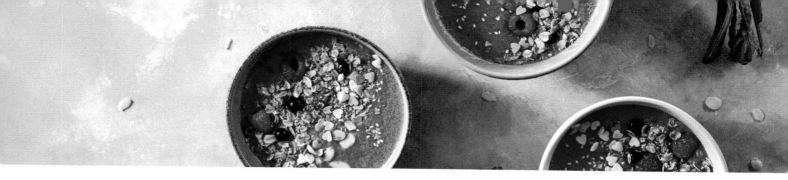

SMOOTHIES

The Heart Beet Blend

A fruity green smoothie with beets and ginger

24 oz water or any nut mylk of your choice
2 small pieces of frozen or fresh beets
1 cup frozen strawberries
1 cup frozen mangoes
1 cup spinach
*1 inch of ginger or 1/4 tsp ginger powder
(optional)

The Power Blend

A delicious green smoothie with extra brotein

24 oz water or any nut mylk of your choice
1 cup kale
5 frozen bananas
1 tbsp almond butter
2 tbsp hemp seeds

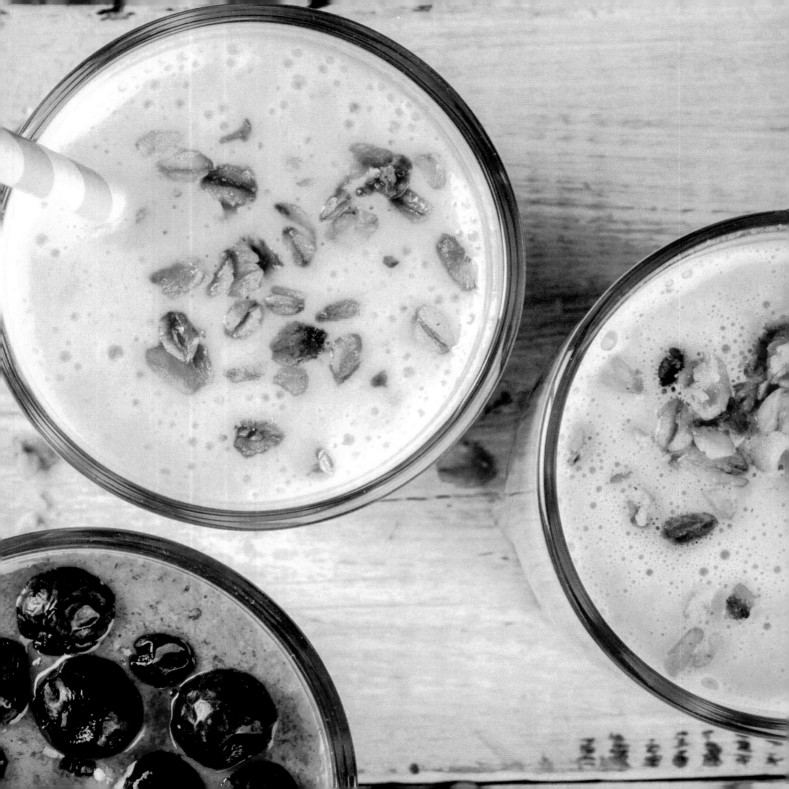

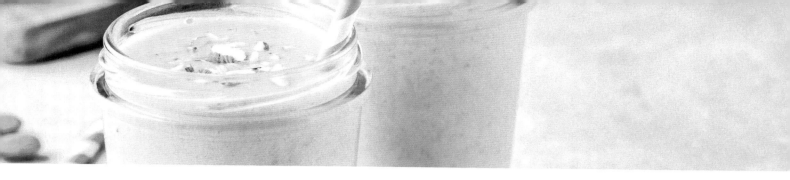

SMOOTHIES

The Synchronicity Blend

A decadent almond butter and jelly smoothie

24 oz water or any nut mylk of your choice
1 cup of spinach
1 cup frozen blueberries
1/2 cup frozen strawberries
5 frozen bananas
2 tbsp almond butter

The Gratitude Blend

Peaches and Creamy Smoothie

24 oz water or any nut mylk of your choice
5 frozen bananas
1 cup frozen peaches
1/2 cup frozen mangoes
1/4 tsp cinnamon

*Add 2 medjool dates if you'd like it extra sweet (optional)

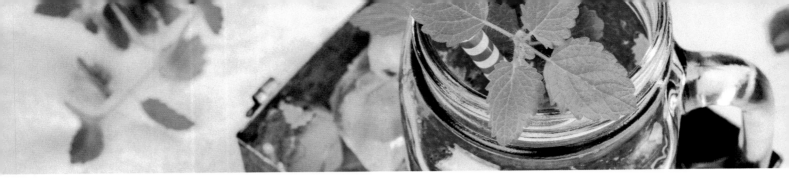

SMOOTHIES

The Miracle Blend
A berry-packed refreshing treat

24 oz water or any nut mylk of your choice
5 frozen bananas
1 cup frozen strawberries
1/2 cup fresh or frozen blackberries
1/2 cup fresh or frozen blueberries

*you can also simply add 2 cups of mixed berries

Pina Colada
So delicious you'll think you're in the tropics!

24 oz water or any nut mylk of your choice
1/2 cup fresh or frozen pineapple
3 frozen bananas
1 orange (peeled and seeded)
1/4 cup young Thai coconut meat (or 1/4 cup shredded coconut)

Chai Dream
A delicious morning or afternoon pick me up!

24 oz water or any nut mylk of your choice
5 frozen bananas
1 tbsp chai mix
2 medjool dates (optional)

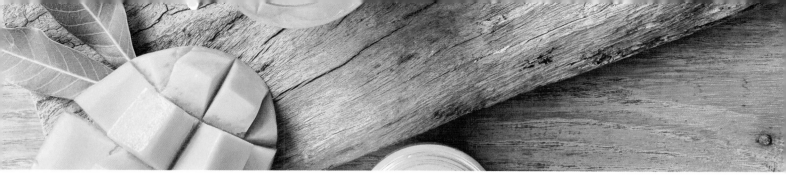

SMOOTHIES

Banana Mango Sunshine

20 oz freshly made orange juice
5 frozen bananas
1 and 1/2 cups frozen mango

Chocolate Carob Smoothie

24 oz water or any nut mylk of your choice
5 frozen bananas
6 dates (de-pitted and soaked for 10 min if firm)
2 tbsp raw carob
1" vanilla bean

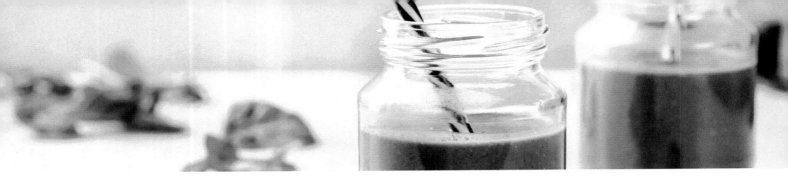

SMOOTHIES

Spirulina Smoothie

20 oz freshly made apple juice or water
1 cup frozen mango
5 frozen bananas
1 tbsp spirulina

Strawberry Kiwi Smoothie

24 oz water or any nut mylk of your choice
1 cup fresh or frozen strawberries
3 golden kiwis, peeled
5 frozen bananas
2 medjool dates (optional)

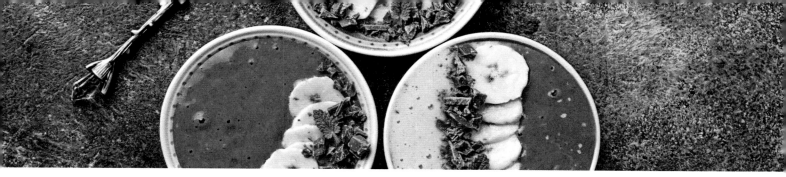

SMOOTHIE BOWLS

Refreshing Mint Chip

1/2 cup water or any nut mylk of your choice
5 frozen bananas
6 drops peppermint spirits or 1/2 tsp peppermint extract
1 medjool date (optional)
Blend – then add 1/4 cup cacao nibs and blend for 5 seconds

Toppings: sliced bananas, shredded coconut, cacao nibs, bananas, and fresh mint

Optional: add 2 tbsp and 2 additional dates cacao to blender to make it a chocolate mint chip smoothie bowl

Chocolate Heaven

1/2 cup water or any nut mylk of your choice
5 frozen bananas
3 tbsp cacao powder
2 tbsp almond butter

Toppings: fresh banana slices, cacao nibs, almond butter, and shredded coconut

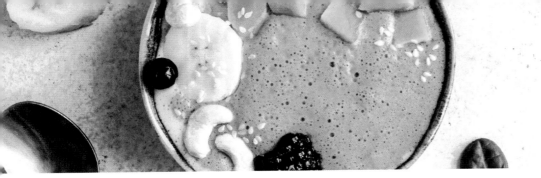

SMOOTHIE BOWLS

Coconut Vanilla Bliss

1/2 cup water or any nut mylk of your choice
2 tbsp hemp seeds
5 frozen bananas
1/2 cup shredded coconut
1" vanilla

Toppings: sliced bananas, shredded coconut, and mulberries

Green Gratitude

1/2 cup water or any nut mylk of your choice
1 cup spinach
5 frozen bananas
1/2 cup frozen mango
1/2 cup fresh or frozen pineapple

Toppings: hemp seeds, berries, and sliced bananas

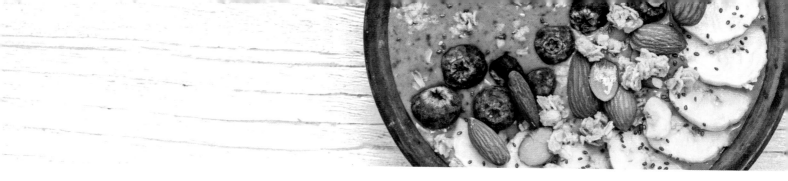

SMOOTHIE BOWLS

Pink Peace

1/2 cup water or any nut mylk of your choice
1 pack frozen pitaya
1/2 cup strawberries
5 frozen bananas
1/2 cup mango

Toppings: sliced bananas, blueberries, kiwi, coconut chips, and/or granola

Chocolate Heaven

1/2 cup water or any nut mylk of your choice
5 frozen bananas
3 tbsp cacao powder
3 medjool dates
3 tbsp almond butter

Toppings: sliced bananas, cacao nibs, almond butter, shredded coconut

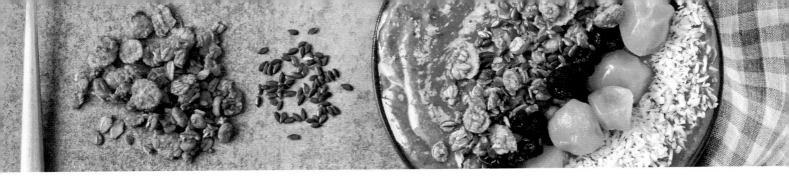

SMOOTHIE BOWLS

Acai Spirulina

1/2 cup water or any nut mylk of your choice
5 frozen bananas
1 cup frozen mixed berries
1 slightly defrosted Acai Packet
1/4 tsp spirulina

Add 2 medjool dates if you'd like it extra sweet!

Toppings: granola, fresh blueberries, mangoes, shredded coconut and dulce de leche (see my recipe in this book!)

Acai PB&J

1/2 cup water or any nut mylk of your choice
1 slightly defrosted Acai packet
1 Tbsp almond butter
1 cup frozen strawberry
4 frozen bananas

Toppings: granola, sliced banana, and nut butter of your choice

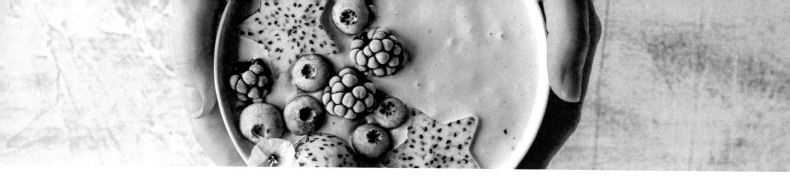

SMOOTHIE BOWLS

Blue Spirulina Dream Bowl

1/2 cup water or any nut mylk of your choice
5 frozen bananas
1 cup frozen mangoes
1 Tbsp blue spirulina

Top with frozen blueberries, blackberries, white dragon fruit, and shredded coconut.

Pink Lemonade Smoothie Bowl

1/2 cup water or any nut mylk of your choice
5 frozen bananas
1/3 cup frozen strawberries
1/3 cup frozen raspberries
2 Tbsp lemon juice

Top with shredded coconut and fresh strawberries.

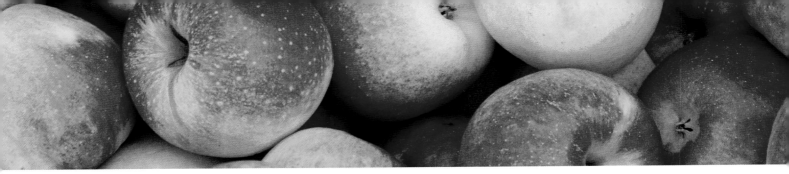

BREAKFAST

Raw Vegan Cereal

Ingredients

Add any (or all!) of the following to a large bowl:

- Apple (chopped into small cubes)
- Banana (sliced)
- Fresh or defrosted frozen berries: blueberries, strawberries, blackberries, and/or raspberries
- Raisins, dates (de-pitted and chopped into small pieces), mulberries, dried coconut and/or any other dried fruit you like.
- Cinnamon (optional)

Add mylk of your choice (I use banana mylk or hemp mylk)

- To make hemp mylk, simply blend 2 cups water, 1" of fresh vanilla bean (optional) and 2 tbsp hemp seeds and 2 dates!
- To make banana mylk simply blend 2 frozen bananas and 2 cups water, 1" of fresh vanilla bean (optional) and 1 date (optional)

Instructions:

1. Chop up the apple and slice banana
2. Add any (or all!) of the above ingredients into a cereal bowl
3. Pour in mylk and viola!

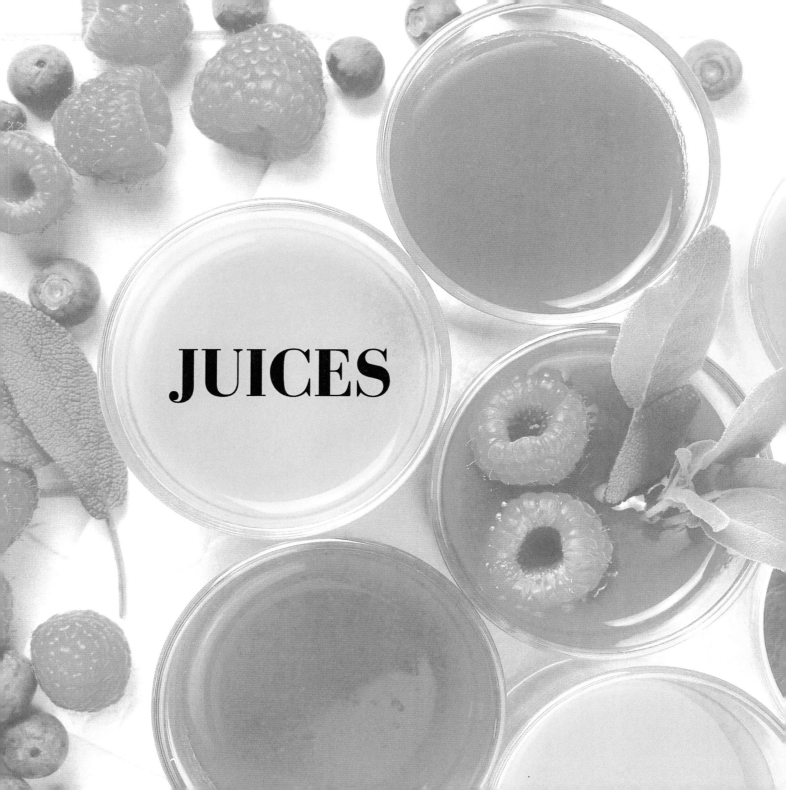

JUICES

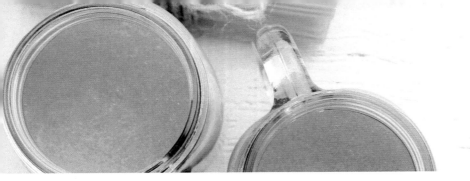

JUICES

Creativity Juice

1/2 a pineapple
3 apples
2 kiwis
1 inch of ginger
1 beet

Abundance Juice

1 beet
4 apples
4 carrots
1/2 a lemon

Resilience Juice

4 carrots
6 apples
1/2 inch fresh turmeric
1 inch fresh ginger

My All-Time Favorite Fruit Juice

1 pint of Strawberries
6 Navel Oranges
1 Pineapple

Candy Apple Juice

6 large apples (I like fuji)
2 inches fresh ginger
1 inch fresh turmeric
2 lemons

Simple Powerful Elixir

5 carrots
1 apple
1 entire bunch of parsley

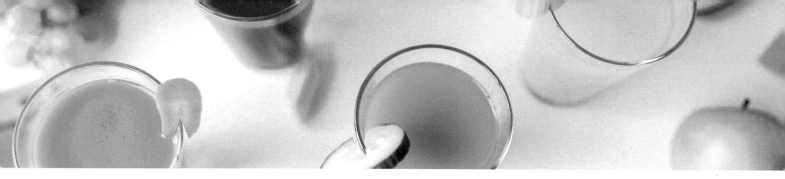

JUICES

Glow with the Flow Juice

4 apples
1 cucumber
2 cups spinach
1/2 a pineapple
3 kiwis

My Favorite Green Juice

5 apples
1 cucumber
1/2 fennel
2 cups spinach
1 lemon

Determination Juice

1/2 bunch of celery
2 cucumbers
1/2 head of romaine
1/2 bunch of parsley
2 cups spinach

Chef Babette's Fav Green Juice

3 green apples
1/2 bunch cilantro
1" ginger
1" turmeric
1 lime

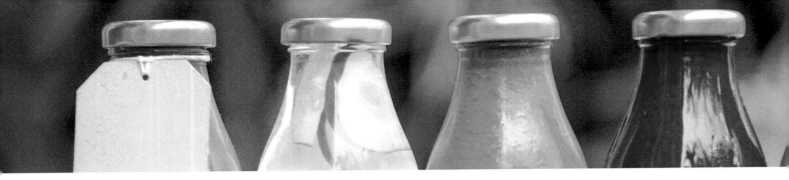

JUICE RECIPES FOR SPECIFIC HEALTH ISSUES

For 30 days...follow a raw or high raw vegan diet, drink one of these juices, eliminate processed foods and dead animal body parts, and watch what happens!

Acne
10 carrots
2 cups of spinach

Anemia
6 large carrots
1 beet
4 cups spinach
1/4 cup watercress

Arthritis
8 large carrots
1 beet
2 cucumbers

Liver Healer
1 beet with the green top
5 apples

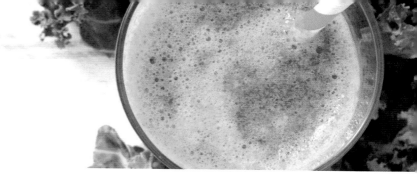

JUICE RECIPES FOR
SPECIFIC HEALTH ISSUES

Diarrhea

4 stalks of celery
1 bulb of fennel
1 bunch of spinach
2 apples

Sinus

6 large carrots
1 bunch of celery
1 handful of parsley

Skin

5 carrots
5 apples
1/2 bunch of celery

Hair Loss

10 carrots
2 cucumbers

SNACKS

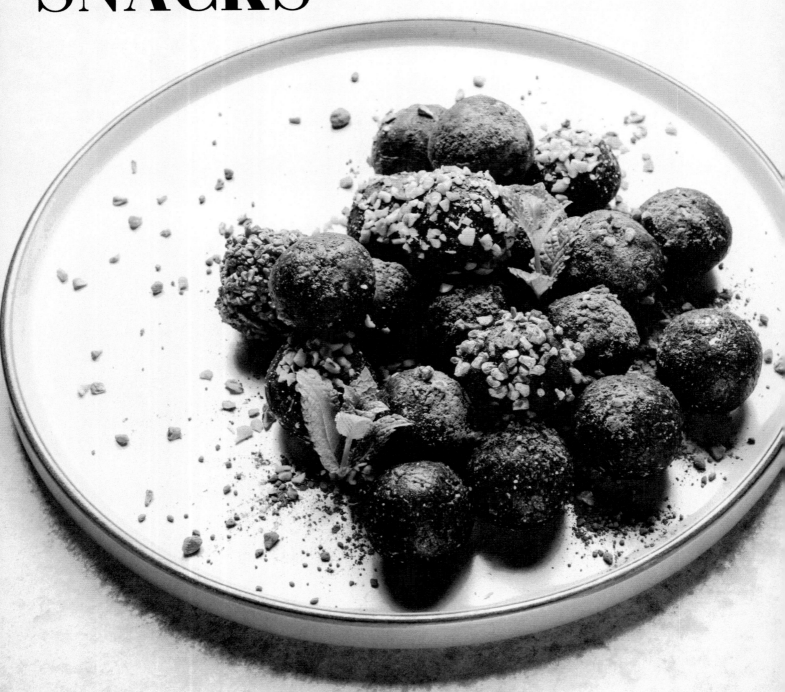

PRO TIP:

The dates and nuts you use make a huge difference in how good your raw food recipes will taste!

I have ZERO affiliation with these companies but I personally like to get AMAZING freshly picked organic dates from **www.BautistaOrganicDates.com**

and I get my nuts from **www.LivingNutz.com**

(They are raw, organic, pre-soaked and sprouted and they taste so much better and fresher than store bought nuts! I find they also digest better too!)

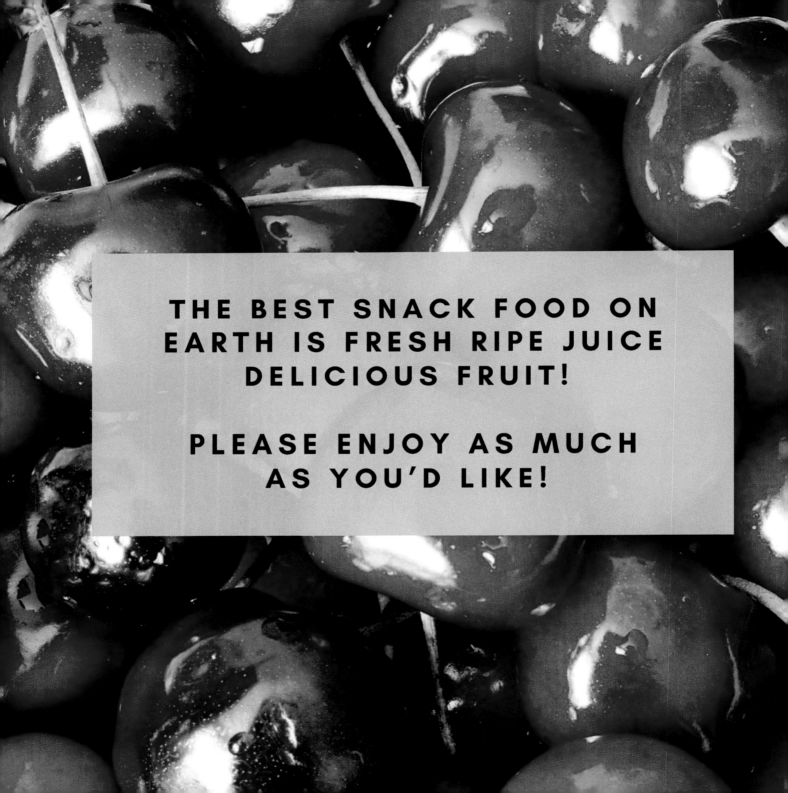

THE BEST SNACK FOOD ON EARTH IS FRESH RIPE JUICE DELICIOUS FRUIT!

PLEASE ENJOY AS MUCH AS YOU'D LIKE!

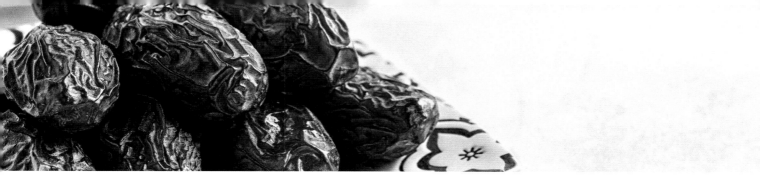

SWEET SNACKS

Chocolate Date Bites | AKA The Quick Fix

When you have no time but in need of a quick sweet fix!

One of the most simple, quick and delicious treats on earth!

Medjool dates, pitted
Almond, cashew or macadamia nut butter
Cacao nibs or a piece of raw vegan chocolate or finely chopped
pistachios, pecand or almonds
Himilayan pink salt (optional)

Instructions:
Remove pit from date. Place nut butter where pit was. Roll date in
cacao nibs or chopped nuts or place a piece of Hu chocolates on top
of nut butter. If you want a sweet and salty fix, sprinkle a little
Himalayan pink salt on top. Yum!

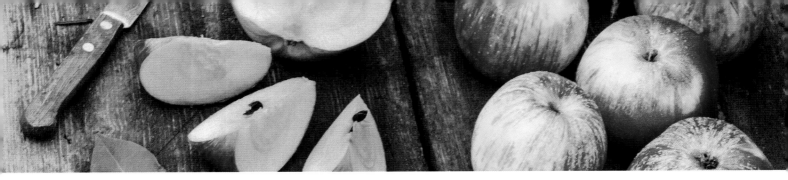

SWEET SNACKS

Caramel with Apple Slices

Perfect to swirl into nice cream or use for dipping apples, bananas, pears, etc

10 medjool dates, pitted
1/2 cup water
1/4 tsp pink salt
1" vanilla bean

Instructions:
1. Add dates, 1/3 cup water, salt and the inside of the vanilla into a blender or food processor.
2. Blend on low for 10-20 seconds, then slowly turn the blender to the highest speed and blend for an additional 30-90 seconds.
3. Add more water as needed since dates will vary in size and dryness. You want a sticky and somewhat thick consistency, similar to a very thick and sticky applesauce. When done, the sauce should be silky smooth with no chunks.
4. Serve right away or store in the fridge until ready to use.
5. Serve over nice cream, as a sweetener, put in milkshakes and smoothies, over raw vegan cheesecake, or simply have with fruit or even with celery for a salty and sweet treat! It's so darn delicious that you can honestly dip just about ANYTHING into it and it will be incredible!

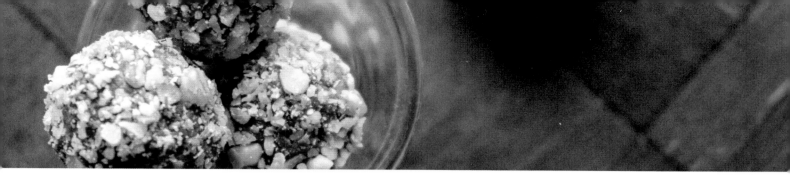

SWEET SNACKS

Cinnamon Bun Balls

½ cup walnuts
5 medjool dates, pitted
3 tablespoons ground cinnamon
1 teaspoon ground cardamom
1 tablespoon finely chopped walnuts, or to taste

Instructions:
Blend 1/2 cup walnuts, dates, cinnamon, and cardamom together in a blender until almost smooth. Roll mixture into little balls. Place finely chopped walnuts in a shallow bowl and roll the balls in walnuts to coat if desired. Store them in refrigerator.

Walnut Fudge Truffles

1 cup walnuts
1 cup medjool dates
2 Tbsp raw cacao
2 Tbsp cacao nibs

Instructions:
Combine all ingredients (except cacao nibs) in food processor When mixed thoroughly, add in cacao nibs at last minute and pulse. Roll into balls. Store in fridge or freezer!

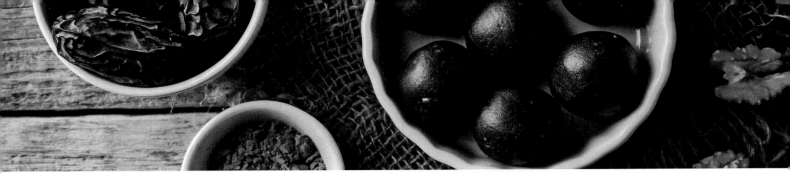

SWEET SNACKS

Energy Balls

If you're out of dates or dates are not your thing, these are super yummy and date-free!

1 cup brazil nuts
1 cup hazelnuts
1 fresh persimmon (extremely ripe and gooey)
1/4 cup raisins
1-2 Tbsp maple syrup

Instructions:
Blend ingredients in food processor until thoroughly mixed. Roll mixture into small balls. Finish by rolling in carob powder or coconut flakes.

Fat Free Date Balls

1 cup mulberries
1 cup dates
1/2 cup dried figs
4 Tbsp cacao powder

Instructions:
Blend ingredients in food processor until thoroughly mixed. Roll mixture into small balls. Finish by rolling in carob powder or coconut flakes.

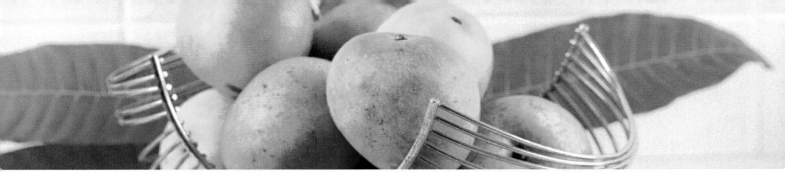

SWEET SNACKS

Ginger Mango Cupcakes

(more than 5 ingredients I know! but its so yummy I had to include it :)

Crust:
1/2 cup almonds
1/2 cup sunflower seeds
6 medjool dates, pitted
1/2 tsp cinnamon
1/4 tsp Himalayan pink salt

Mango layer:
1 cup cashews
2 Tbsp maple syrup
1 large mango (super ripe)
1 tsp fresh ginger
1 Tbsp lime juice
1/4 tsp cinnamon

Instructions:
Mix all crust ingredients in a food processor or high speed blender until fully combined. Place into circular cookie cutters or in cupcake pan lined with baking cups. Blend all mango layer ingredients in a high speed powered blender. Pour on top. Top cupcakes with shredded coconut, lime zest and or chocolate. Place into refrigerator to set for at least 20 min.

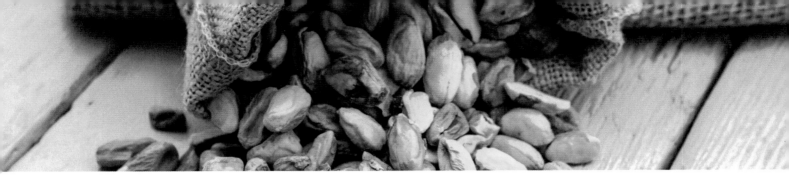

SWEET SNACKS

Pistachio Balls

1 cups pistachios (not soaked)
1 cup golden raisins
1 cup dates
1/2 tsp nutmeg

Instructions:
Blend in a food processor until thoroughly mixed.
Take a Tbsp of the mixture and roll into a ball.
Place balls in freezer or roll balls in carob powder
or coconut flakes!

Pina Colada Balls

1 cup coconut flakes
1 cup macadamia nuts
1 cup dried pineapple, (chopped and soaked for 30 min)
1/2 cup golden raisins
1 tsp vanilla extract

Instructions:
Blend in a food processor until mixed thoroughly. Take a
Tbsp of the mixture and roll into a ball. Place balls in
freezer or roll balls in coconut flakes!

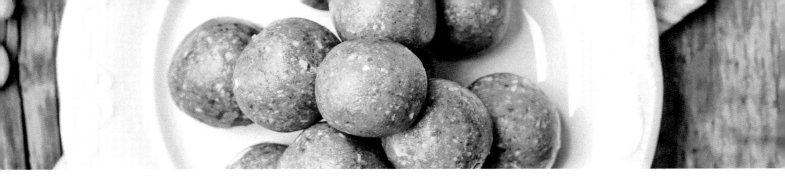

SWEET SNACKS

Cashew Mulberry Balls

1 cup cashews
1/2 cup mulberries
1 tsp vanilla extract
1 Tbsp carob powder
1/6 tsp Himalayan salt (optional)

Almond Butter Balls

1/2 cup almond butter
20 medjool dates
1 cup almonds, cashews or sunflower seeds
1/2 cup coconut flakes
1/2 tsp cinnamon
a pinch of Himalayan salt (optional)

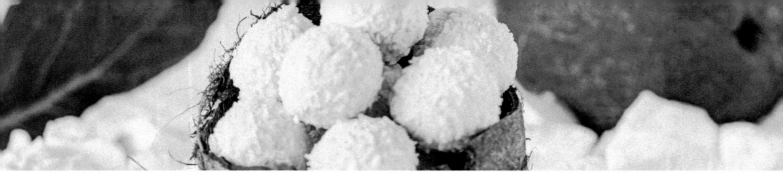

SWEET SNACKS

Vanilla Coconut Carob Bites

1/4 cup cashews
1/4 cup dates
1/4 cup carob powder
1/4 cup shredded coconut
1" scrape vanilla bean
water

Instructions:
Roll into balls. Place on parchment paper and roll in shredded coconut. Freeze for at least 20 minutes before serving.

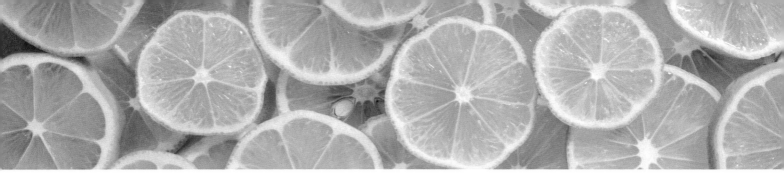

SAVORY + SPICY SNACKS

Celery Date Delights

Celery
Dates

Another super simple delicious treat is to take a few celery stalks and place pitted dates (any kind) inside of the celery. This seems so simple but try it! It's such an easy healthy and yummy salty and sweet treat!

Spicy Lime Balls

1/4 cup dates
2 cups almonds
1/2 cup cashews
1 lime (juice + zest)
1/2 small chili pepper
minced 1 teaspoon ginger

Instructions:
Blend all ingredients (without adding any water) in food processor, about 2 minutes. Shape into balls, and store in the refrigerator at least 2 hours before consuming.

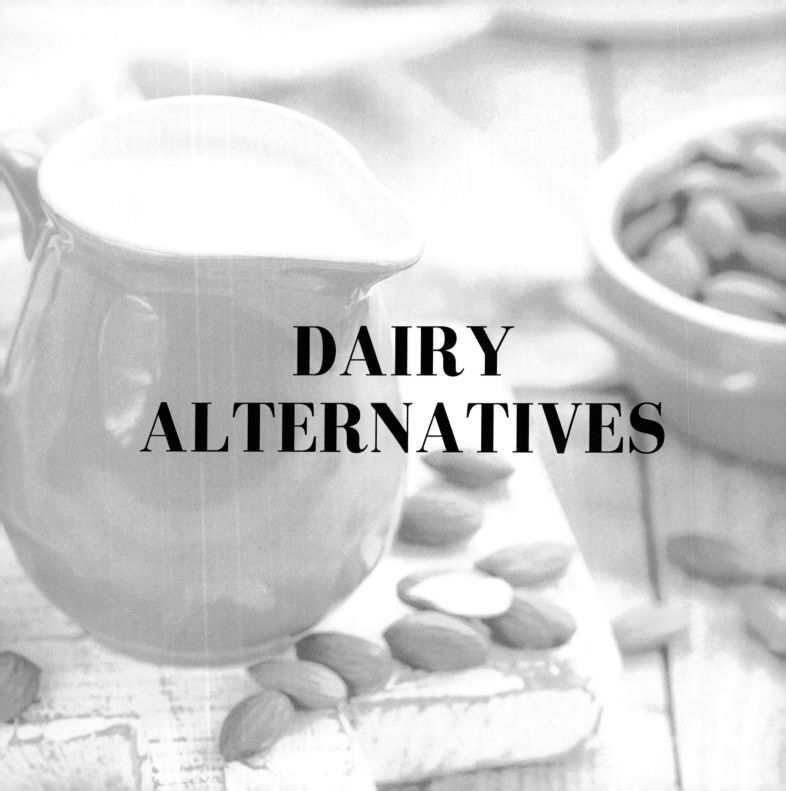

DAIRY ALTERNATIVES

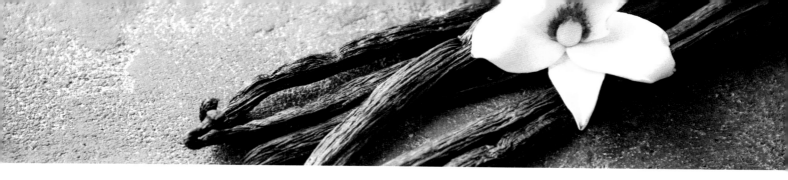

PUDDING

Vanilla Pudding

1 cup water or nut mylk of choice
1 TBPS hemp seeds
2 ripe bananas
6 dates (soaked for 10 min)
1/2" freshly scraped vanilla bean
1/4 tsp nutmeg (or less)

Blend in high speed blender

Coconut Strawberry Pudding

1 coconut (meat + water)
1 cup of fresh strawberries
4 dates

Blend in high speed blender

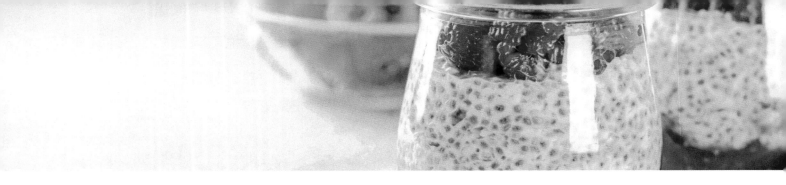

CHIA PUDDING

Chia Pudding

4 Tbsp chia seeds
1 cup fresh almond mylk*
1/2" of freshly scraped vanilla bean (optional)

*feel free to use ANY type of nut mylk including coconut, cashew, hemp mylk, etc. If nut mylk is unsweetened then blend it FIRST with 2 pitted medjool dates or you can use 1/2 Tablespoon maple syrup)

Toppings of choice: fresh berries or other fruit, granola, nut butter, etc

Instructions:
In a bowl or mason jar, stir together chia seeds, nut mylk and maple syrup and vanilla, if you so wish. If you're using a mason jar, you can put the lid on and shake the mixture to combine everything.

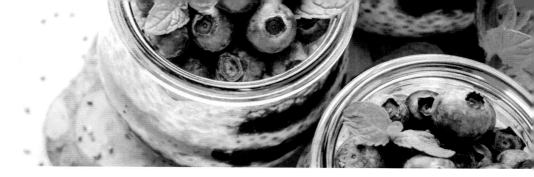

CHIA PUDDING

Once the chia pudding mixture is well combined, let it sit for 5 minutes, give it another stir/shake to break up any clumps of chia seeds, cover and put the mixture in the fridge to "set" for 1-2 hours or overnight (best)

The chia pudding should be nice and thick, not liquidy. If it's not thick enough, just add more chia seeds (about 1 Tablespoon), stir and refrigerate for another 30 minutes or so.

Chia pudding can be stored for up to 5-7 days in an airtight container in the refrigerator.

I LOVE to make a berry jam to stir into my chia pudding Not only is it delicious but it makes the chia pudding into a GORGEOUS color! ! Plus, it's so simple to make, you will LOVE it! (recipe on next page)

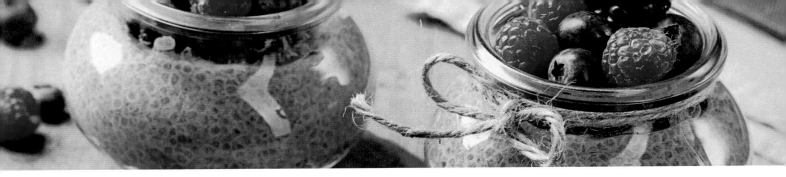

MIXED BERRY JAM

2 cups mixed berries (for this recipe I like to purchase my berries frozen and defrost them)

2-6 dates (depending on how sweet you want it)

Instructions:

Place berries and dates in a high speed blender. Use tamper and blend until you've reached desired consistency. Test out jam's sweetness by starting with only two dates in the blender. Add more if jam is not sweet.

You don't have to use mixed berries. You can also simply use 1 type of fruit + dates. You can use strawberries, blueberries, mangoes, etc

If you HATE seeds in your jam, do not use raspberries or blackberries.

If you LOVE seeds in your jam then you can add chia seeds at the end and pulse for a few seconds.

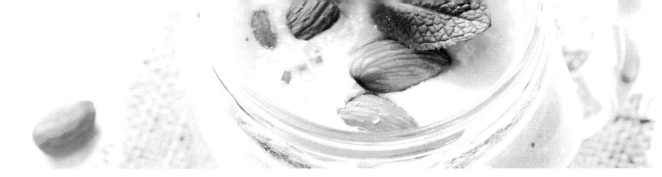

NUT MYLKS

Almond Mylk

1 cup almonds (soaked in water overnight in refridgerator)
3 cups water
2 dates

Combine all ingredients in a blender. Once blended, strain through a nut mylk bag or very fine strainer into another container. Store in the refrigerator where it will keep 4 to 5 days.

These directions can be followed to make all kinds of other nut mylks including but not limited to: cashew mylk, hazelnut mylk, walnut mylk, pecan mylk, brazil nut mylk, etc.

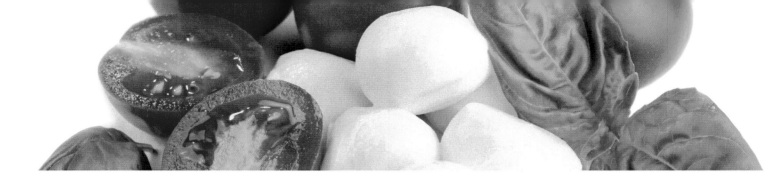

CHEESE

Mozzarella Cheese

1 cup of cashews (soaked over night)
1 tbsp lemon juice
2 tbsp psyllium husk *(this is the one weird ingredients in this book – sorry– you can find at a health food store or order on amazon)*
1 pinch of garlic powder

Blend all the ingredients in a high speed blender (without the soaking water). Sometimes it is necessary to add a bit more psyllium husk, sometimes you may need to add a tiny bit of water, just enough to create a thick, creamy consistency. With wet hands form little Mozzarella cheese balls and let them thicken up in the fridge over night.

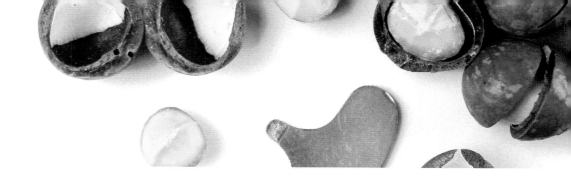

CHEESE

Cheesy Yumminess

(AMAZING on zucchini pasta or as a dressing!)

1 and 1/2 cups cashews soaked for at least two hours and drained
Juice of 1 large lemon
2-3 tablespoons clove garlic
3 tablespoons non fortified nutritional yeast
1/2 tsp Himalayan pink salt (optional)
1 cup water (or more depending on desired consistency)

Combine all ingredients in food processor or blender and blend until the mixture is smooth.

Simple and Easy Parmesan Cheese

1/2 a cup brazil nuts
1-2 cloves garlic
1/2 tsp Himalayan pink salt (optional)

Place brazil nuts, garlic and salt into a food processor and pulse until it looks like parmesan!

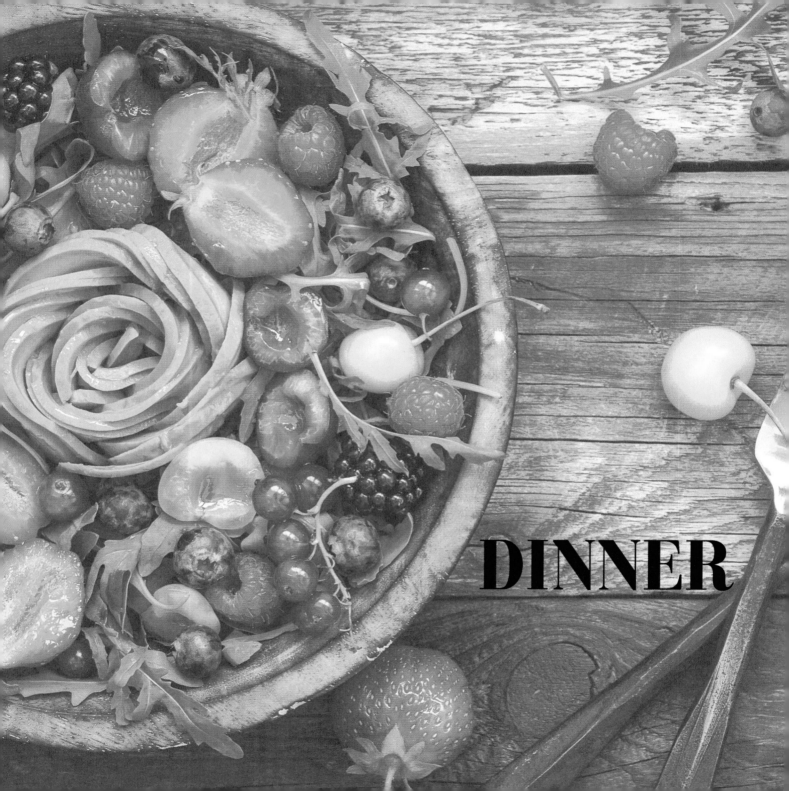

DINNER

PRO TIP

EACH DINNER ENTRÉE SHARED HERE SHOULD BE ENJOYED WITH A LARGE RAW SALAD WITH AN AMAZING HOMEMADE DRESSING!

IF YOU DO NOT CONSUME LARGE ENOUGH QUANTITIES OF FRUIT AND VEGETABLES THEN YOU WILL FOR SURE BE CRAVING AND DESIRING UNHEALTHY AND PROCESSED FOOD!

IF YOU ARE CRAVING PROCESSED FOOD – YOU ARE NOT EATING ENOUGH FRUIT!

IF YOU ARE CRAVING SALT – YOU ARE NOT EATING ENOUGH VEGETABLES!

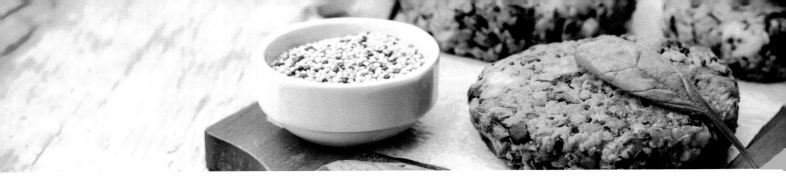

BURGERS

Quick Easy Raw Burger

1/2 cup sunflower seeds (soak for 20 min then rinsed)
1 cup pecans (soaked for 20 min then rinsed)
2 cups cabbage
2 avocados

Instructions:
Combine all ingredients in food processor and pulse until the mixture is thoroughly mixed. Shape into patties and serve on top of salad or on lettuce leaves with tomato slices and a creamy dressing!

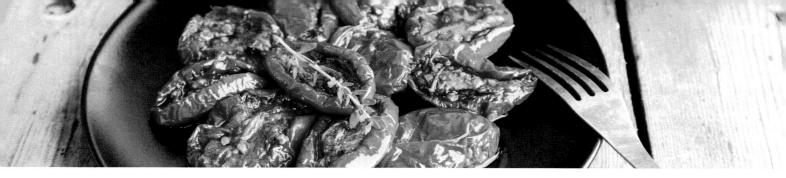

TACO SALAD

Taco Meat

1 cup walnuts
1/2 cup sun-dried tomato halves well-packed,
soaked for at least 2 hours and drained
1/2 tsp ground cumin
1/4 tsp garlic powder
a pinch chili powder or cayanne pepper (or more
if you like it hot)
1/8 tsp Himalayan salt (optional)

Instructions:
Process all of the walnut taco meat ingredients
in a food processor until well combined, but still
chunky.

Sour Cream

1 cup cashews, (soaked 1 hour)
1/4 cup lemon juice
1/4 tsp salt
3 cup water

Instructions:
Blend all of the cashew sour cream
ingredients in a blender until smooth
and creamy.

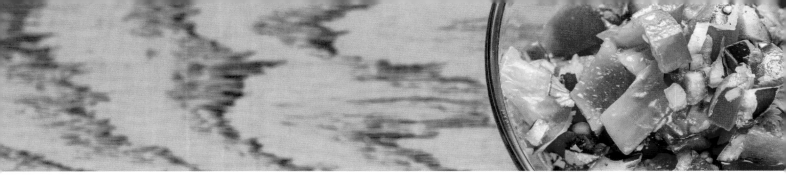

TACO SALAD

Guacamole

1 avocado
1 tsp lemon or lime juice
1 tomato (finely chopped)
1/4 cup cilantro (finely chopped)
1/4 tsp Himalayan Pink Salt (optional)

Salsa

5 tomatoes (I like to use Roma)
1/2 cup cilantro (finely chopped)
juice of 1 lemon
2 green onions
1 red pepper (finely chopped)

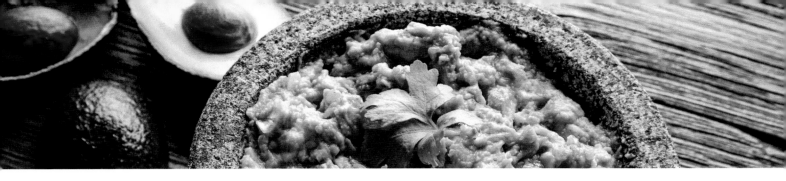

TACO SALAD

Complete Taco Salad Ingredients:

3 cups romaine lettuce
1-2 cucumbers, diced
2 spring onions or 1/4 of a red onion
1/2 cup corn (if desired)

Add:
Guacamole or simple 1/2 an avocado
Salsa
Cashew Sour Cream
Walnut Taco Meat

RAW VEGAN SUSHI WRAPS

Nori sheets (purchase the large Nori sheet with no salt or oil added. Feel free to use the raw or toasted ones, whichever you prefer. Trust me, consuming a few healthy non-raw things once in a while will not ruin your raw vegan lifestyle or health!)

Inside - place any of the following thinly sliced ingredients:

mango
red cabbage
green onions
carrots
cilantro
sprouts
cucumbers
avocado

Once ingredients are on sheet, roll up nori sheets! You can cut them with a very sharp knife if desired. Be sure to not get nori sheets wet or they will not roll!

Option: feel free to add one of the patès, dips or dressings in this recipe book to the nori sheet first before placing ingredients on top.

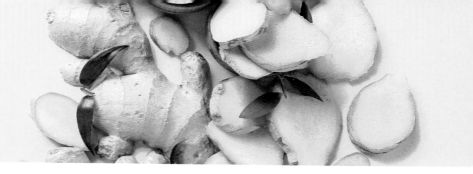

RAW VEGAN SUSHI WRAPS

Nori Wraps Dipping Sauce:

1/4 cup maple syrup
juice from 1/2 a lime
splash of coconut aminos
1/4 tsp grated ginger or ginger powder
a dash of cayenne pepper

Instructions:
Simply whisk sauce in bowl. Use this sauce or ANY other
sauce that you love!

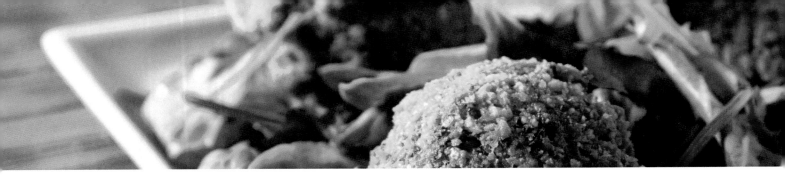

RAW VEGAN FALAFEL WRAPS

There are 7 ingredients in the falafels (I know! I know! :)
but these are so good I HAD to include them!

Falafels

3/4 cup sunflower seeds
2 cups chopped carrots
1/2 cup cilantro
1 tsp lime juice
1/2 tsp coriander seeds
1/2 tsp cumin seeds
1/2 cup chopped green onions

Instructions:
Place ingredients into food processor and process until all ingredients are thoroughly mixed but stop before over mixing. Mixture should stick together when rolled!

Spread mixture onto collard, cabbage (my fav to use!) or romaine wraps with:

spinach
mixed greens
romaine
tomato
cucumber
peppers
sprouts
and/or whatever else you'd like!

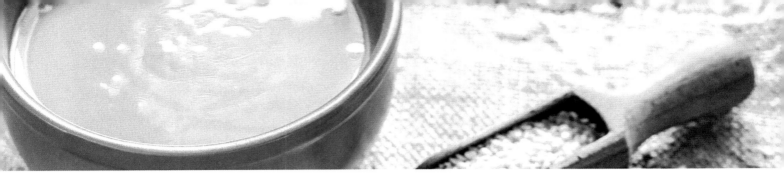

RAW VEGAN FALAFEL WRAPS

Or you can roll the falafel mixture into balls!

Take a large piece of purple Cabbage and place butter lettuce inside. Add tomatoes, cilantro and a few falafel balls.

Serve either version of the falafel wrap with a simple tahini sauce:

1/2 tbsp tahini (or 1/2 cup sesame seeds)
1 tbsp water
1 tbsp lime juice

Instructions:
Simply whisk together ingredients with a fork.

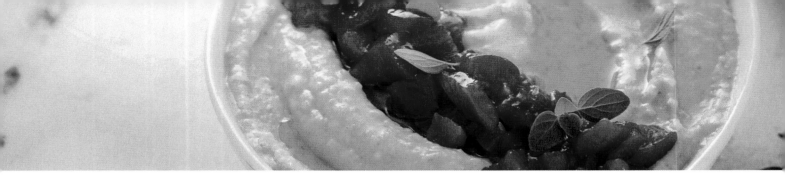

VEGGIES WITH HUMMUS

Cut up slices of cucumbers, peppers (red and orange only), zucchini, celery, romaine lettuce, etc. Place on a plate.

Raw Vegan Red Pepper Hummus

2 red peppers
1 small zucchini
1/3 cup pumpkin seeds
1 tbsp fresh lemon juice
1 clove garlic
1/2 tsp Himalayan pink salt

Instructions:
Place all ingredients in a food processor, or high-speed blender, and blend on high until smooth. If it is not thick enough, add 2 more Tbsp of pumpkins seeds and blend again until smooth.

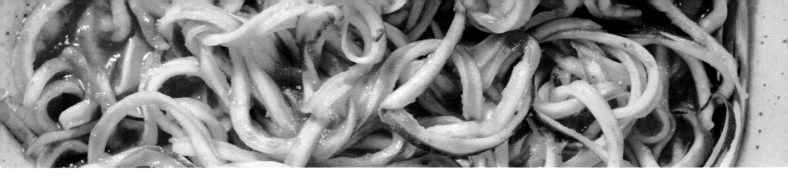

ZUCCHINI NOODLES WITH MARINARA SAUCE

Pasta

4 medium to large green zucchinis

Raw Vegan Marinara Sauce

1 lb. tomatoes (roma, grape or cherry, on the vine, etc)
1 cup sun-dried tomatoes (not in oil)
1 clove garlic (or 1 teaspoon garlic powder)
2 green onions
1/2 cup herbs (cilantro, parsley or basil)

Spirulize the zucchini (first cut off tips of zucchini and if desired, soak in warm water)

For the sauce:
Start with softening the sun-dried tomatoes. Do this by placing them in a small bowl of warm, not boiling, water, and let soak for about 20 minutes. Drain water. Once tomatoes are ready, place all the ingredients into a food processor or blender, and blend until mixture is fairly smooth. You can also leave it a little chunky if you like. Taste for flavor adding more of anything you like.

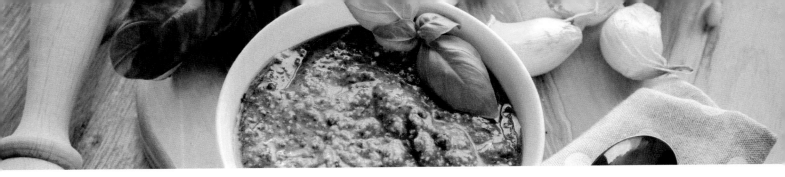

ZUCCHINI NOODLES WITH PESTO

Pasta

4 medium to large green zucchinis and/or cucumbers

Raw Vegan Pesto

1/2 cup pine nuts
1 tbsp lemon juice
1 tbsp nutritional yeast
1 cup fresh parsley
1 cup fresh basil

1 clove garlic (optional)
1 tsp Himalayan Pink Salt (optional)

Spirulize the zucchini (first cut off tips of zucchini and if desired, soak in warm water)

For the sauce:
Combine all ingredients in a blender or food processor and blend until smooth. Add water as needed!

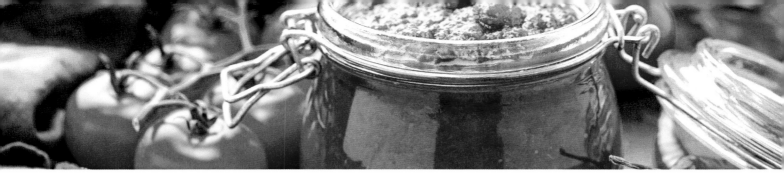

SOUPS | SAUCES

Creamy Tomato Soup | Tomato Sauce

8 tomatoes
1/2 cup tahini or pine nuts
1/4 cup fresh basil
1 tsp Himalayan pink salt
3 green onions
2 cups water

Instructions:
Combine all ingredients into a blender and blend until you reach desired consistency. Use less water to make a fabulous tomato sauce for zucchini noodles!

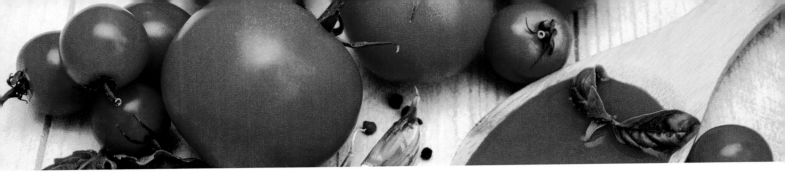

SAUCE

Tomato Basil Sauce

1 cup fresh chopped tomatoes
2 cloves garlic
1/2 cup basil
juice of 1 lemon
3 dates
1 cup sun dried tomatoes

Instructions:
Blend in a high speed powdered blender or food processor until desired consistency.

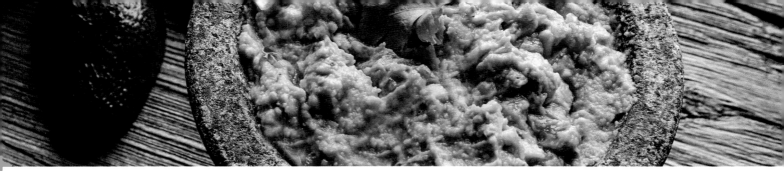

DIPS

I honestly don't eat many salads. Instead I like to make 5 min diners by quickly chopping up cucumbers, peppers, tomatoes, lettuce and dipping them in dressings or dips. Often I make wraps by placing my cut up crudité into lettuce or nori sheets.

Below are some of my all time favorite dips and dressings.

Guacamole

2 avocados
1 tsp lemon or lime juice
1 tomato (finely chopped)
1/4 cup cilantro (finely chopped)
1/4 tsp Himalayan Pink Salt (optional)

Salsa

5 tomatoes
1/2 cup cilantro (finely chopped)
juice of 1 lemon
2 green onions
1 red pepper (finely chopped)

Instructions:
Blend in a high speed powdered blender until desired consistency.

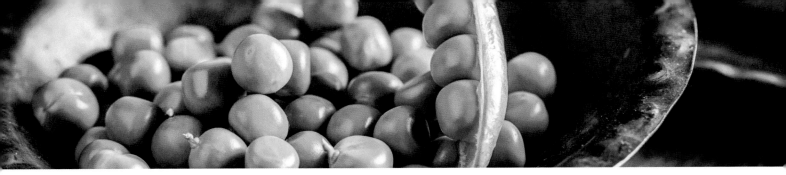

DIPS

Green Pea Guacamole

1 bag of defrosted frozen peas
(approx. 3 cups)
Juice from 1 lime
1 tomato
1/4 cup cilantro
2 cloves garlic

Mayo

1 cup cashews (soaked for 20 min)
2 tsp apple cider vinegar
2 tsp lemon juice
1 or 2 cloves of garlic (depending on your preference)
1/2 cup water
1/4 tsp Himalayan Pink Salt (optional)

Instructions:
Blend in a high speed powdered blender until
desired consistency.

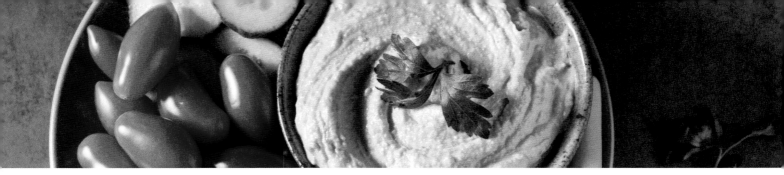

DIPS

Hummus

2 peeled zucchinis
Juice of 1 lemon
2 stalks of green onion
1/2 cup tahini
1 clove garlic

Instructions:
Combine all ingredients in a blender or food processor and blend until smooth. Add a little bit of water as needed!

Low Fat Hummus

2 peeled zucchinis
Juice of 1/2 a lemon
3 stalks of green onion
2 TBSP hemp seeds
1 clove garlic
1/2 cup sun dried tomatoes (rinse 3 times to remove any salt on them)

Instructions:
Combine all ingredients in a blender or food processor and blend until smooth. Add a little bit of water as needed!

Use as a dressing, a dip for wraps or serve with your favorite dipping veggies like mini sweet peppers, carrot, cucumbers, celery, etc

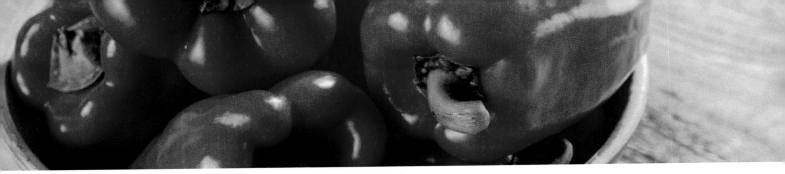

DIPS

Red Pepper Hummus

1 fresh red pepper
1/2 cup pumpkin seeds
1-2 cloves garlic
1/4 cup chopped onions or 3 stalks green onion or 1 TSP onion powder
Juice of 1 lemon

Instructions:
Combine all ingredients in a blender or food processor and blend until smooth. Add a little bit of water as needed!

Pistachio Pesto

2 cups spinach
1 cup basil
1/3 cup pistachios (or sub. with pine nuts, walnuts or cashews)
1/4 cup nutritional yeast
2 cloves garlic
Juice of 1 lemon

Instructions:
Combine all ingredients in a blender or food processor and pulse until blended to desired consistency. Add water as needed.

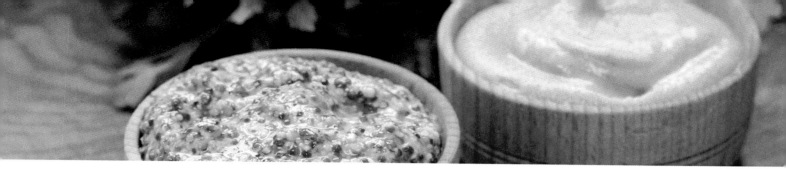

DIPS

Olive Pesto

1/2 cup black olives
1/4 cup fresh basil
1 tbsp lemon juice
1/2 tsp chilli powder
water as needed

Instructions:
Combine all ingredients in a blender or food processor and pulse until blended to desired consistency.

Dijon Mustard Dressing

4 medjool dates (de-pitted)
Juice of 1 lemon
1 Tbsp nutritional yeast
3 Tbsp Dijon mustard (or 1 Tbsp mustard seeds)
2 Tbsp hemp seeds
Splash of coconut aminos (optional)

Instructions:
Combine all ingredients in a blender until blended to desired consistency. Add water as needed.

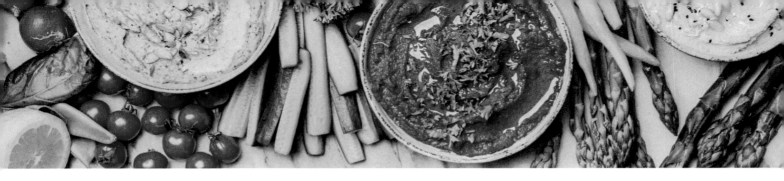

DIPS

Spinach Dip

4 cups fresh spinach
1/2 cup tahini or 1/2 cup sesame seeds
1 tomato
3 tbsp lemon juice
3 green onion stalks

Instructions:
Combine all ingredients in a blender or food processor and blend to desired consistency

Sunflower Dip

1 and 1/2 cups sunflower seeds (soaked overnight then rinsed)
1/2 cup lemon juice
1/4 cup tahini or 1/4 cup sesame seeds
1/4 cup fresh parsley
1 inch fresh ginger

Instructions:
Combine all ingredients in a food processor and puree until desired consistency is reached

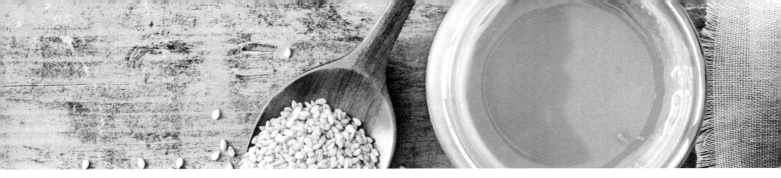

DRESSINGS

Simple Easy Tahini Dressing

1 cup tahini or 1/2 cup sesame seeds
Juice of 1 lemon
1 clove garlic
1/2 cup fresh parsley (or any other herb of choice)
1 date

Instructions:
Combine all ingredients in a blender or food processor and blend until smooth. Add water as needed!

Cheesy Tahini

1 red pepper
3 Tbsp nutritional yeast
1/2 cup tahini
Juice from 1 lemon
1 clove garlic

Instructions:
Combine all ingredients in a blender or food processor and blend until smooth. Add water as needed!

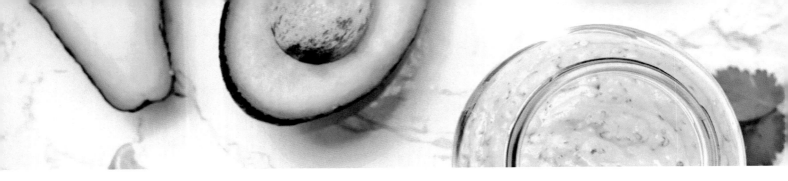

DRESSINGS

Build-Your-Own Avocado Dressing

1/2 an avocado
Juice of 1 lime
2 stalks of celery
Herbs of any choice (parsley, dill or cilantro)
Spices (cayenne, cumin, Italian seasoning, or
nutritional yeast)

Instructions:
Combine all ingredients in a blender or food
processor and blend until smooth. Add water as
needed!

Easiest Dressing In the Universe

1 avocado :)

Instructions:
Massage avocado into salad WITH YOUR HANDS!
Add spices or herbs and finely chopped green
onions if desired. This is such a simple easy dressing
when you are short on ingredients, time or have no
blender available! Perfect for when on the road!
(be sure to have water and napkins readily
available to wash hands after)

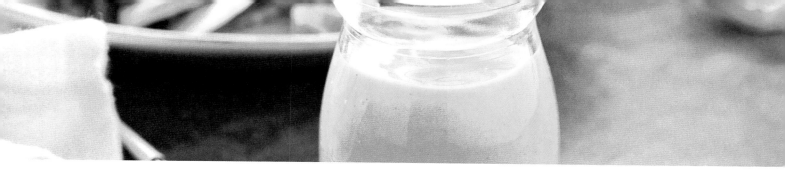

DRESSINGS

Asian Dressing

*I LOVE this dressing over zucchini, carrot and daikon radish noodles,
thinly slices red and orange peppers, cilantro. mmmmm!*

1 cup tahini or 1/2 cup sesame seeds
5 dates (soaked for 10 min)
1 cup orange juice
1/4 cup Nama Shoyu
1/2 inch fresh ginger root

Instructions:

Combine all ingredients in a blender or food processor and blend until
smooth! To make the noodles simply use a spirilizer!

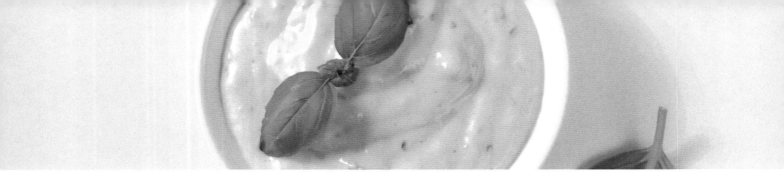

DRESSINGS

Ceasar Dressing

1/2 cup sesame seeds
1 Tbsp dijon mustard
Juice from 1 lemon
3 Tbsp nutritional yeast
1 Tbsp coconut aminos

Instructions:
Blend all ingredients until creamy and smooth

Tomato Mango Sauce
(add more tomatoes if craving salty)

2 medium tomatoes
2 mangoes
Juice from 1/2 a lemon
2-3 green onion stems
1 big handful of dill

Instructions:
Blend all ingredients except dill. Once smooth, add dill and pulse. Service on zucchini noodles or on a salad.

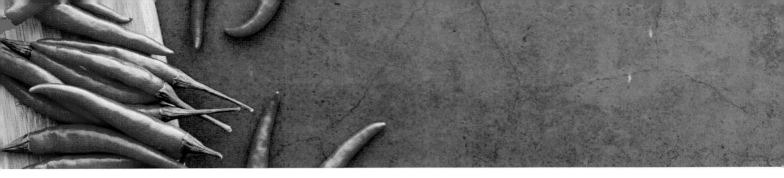

DRESSINGS

Creamy & Spicy Tahini Dressing

1 red pepper
1/2 jalapeño
1/2 lemon
1 clove garlic
1/2 cup sesame seeds
3 dates (optional)

Instructions:
Combine all ingredients in a blender or food processor and blend until smooth. Add water as needed!

Hot Sauce

2 tomatoes
2Tbsp lemon
1 date
1 green onion
Hot pepper to taste

Instructions:
Combine all ingredients in a blender or food processor and blend until smooth. Add water as needed!

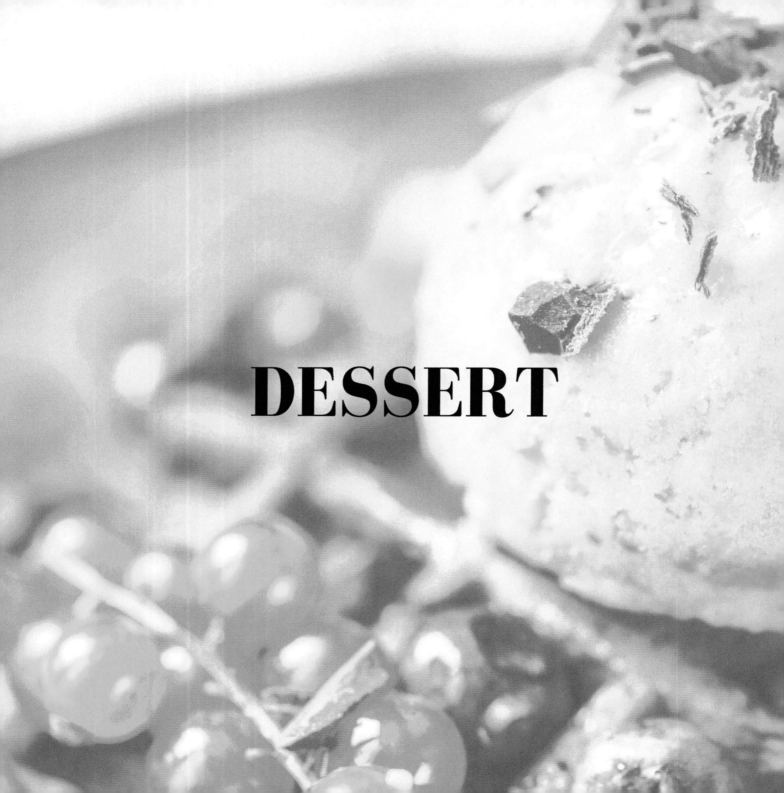

DESSERT

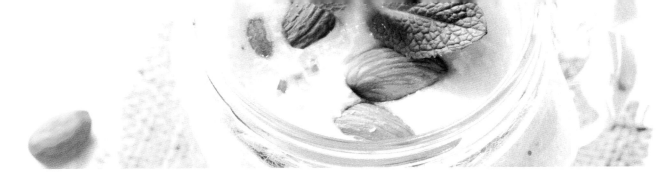

NICE CREAM

Green Nice Cream

5 frozen bananas
1 cup spinach or 1 TSP daily Green Boost
(use my code: Ms.FitVegan for a discount
at checkout)
1 TBSP hemp seeds
1 date
1/8 cup water

Blend using tamper and enjoy!

Pink Fruity Nice Cream
(kids LOVE this one!)

2 frozen bananas
1 cup frozen mangoes
1/2 cup frozen strawberries
1 Tbsp pink dragon fruit powder or 1/2 a
fresh pink dragon fruit
1/4 cup water (omit if using fresh pink
Dragon fruit)

Blend using tamper and enjoy!

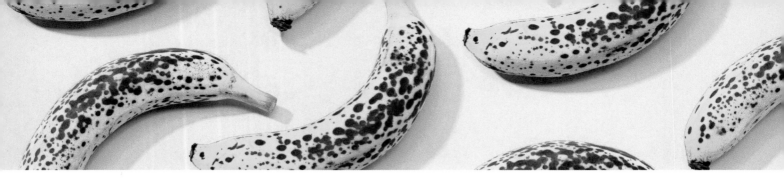

NICE CREAM

Nice Cream Almond Butter Bites
(kids LOVE these!)

(7 ingredients I know – I know BUT YOU HAVE TO MAKE THESE THEY ARE DIVINE!!!)

Crust:
20 medjool dates
1/4 cup almond for coconut flour
2 Tbsp almond butter (or peanut butter)

Nice Cream:
2 frozen bananas
Splash of almond milk
1/4 tsp vanilla powder
1/4 cup cacao nibs or chopped chocolate gems by hu kitchen (I prefer the Hu kitchen chocolates for this recipe)

Instructions:
Blend crust ingredients in a high speed blender or food processor until fully mixed. Take a Tbsp worth of the crust mix and place into a silicon mini muffin pan. Press down until firm. Make nice cream in a high speed powdered blender and mix in chocolate after! Spoon on top of crust. Save some left over crust to crumble on top of nice cream. Place into freezer to set!

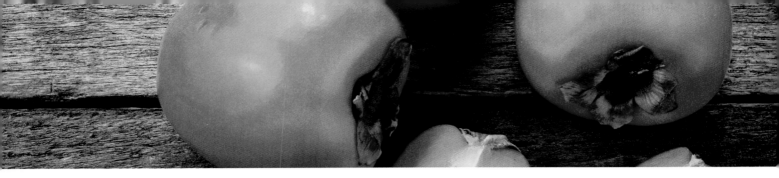

NICE CREAM

The BEST Nice Cream EVER!

5 frozen bananas
1 fresh super ripe Hachiya or Fuyu persimmons
1/2 tsp cinnamon (optional)
1" tsp vanilla bean (optional)

Instructions:

Take the top off and remove any produce sticker on it before placing it into the blender (with skin and all) In the blender add frozen bananas and all other optional ingredients and use tamper to blend on high. You may add 1/2 tsp of pumpkin spice as well if desired. Do not add any water! (unless absolutely necessary)

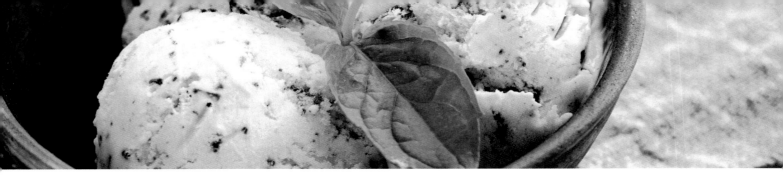

NICE CREAM

Mint Chip Nice Cream

4–5 frozen bananas
2 TBSP cacao nibs
1 drop peppermint spirits or 1 drop peppermint oil
(drop into water first to ensure only 1 drop is used)
1 TBSP hemp seeds or cashews (optional)
2 TBSP water or nut mylk of your choice

Instructions:
Blend everything (except the cacao nibs) in a high speed blender until consistency is almost smooth like ice cream! Stop blender and then add cacao. Then blend for up to 30 seconds or until creamy but chips are still visible. Yummm!

Feel free to add a cup of spinach if you would like it to be green. This will not affect the taste!

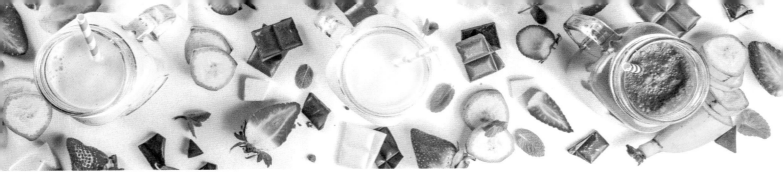

MYLKSHAKES!

Vanilla Mylk Shake

10oz cashew mylk or 1/2 cup cashews + 1 cup water
2 cups frozen banana
1 tsp vanilla extract
2 medjool dates

Strawberry Mylk Shake

10oz cashew mylk or 1/2 cup cashews + 1 cup water
2 cups frozen bananas
1 cup frozen strawberries
2 medjool dates

Chocolate Mylk Shake

10oz cashew mylk or 1/2 cup cashews + 1 cup water
2 cups frozen bananas
3 tbsp cacao powder
3 medjool dates

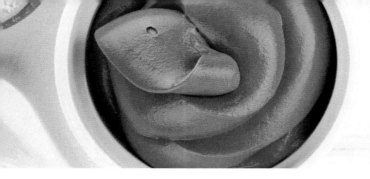

DULCE DE LECHE

Swirl into Nice Cream or dip apples or frozen bananas into this delicious treat!

Step 1: Make the Mylk

Ingredients:
1/2 cup hazelnuts
2 barhi dates

Blend in a high speed blender and then strain through a nut mylk bag

Step 2: Make the Dulce De Leche

Ingredients:
1/2 to 1 cup hazelnut mylk
1 cup barhi dates

Blend in a high speed blender until thick and creamy. Add mylk as needed (up to 1 cup)

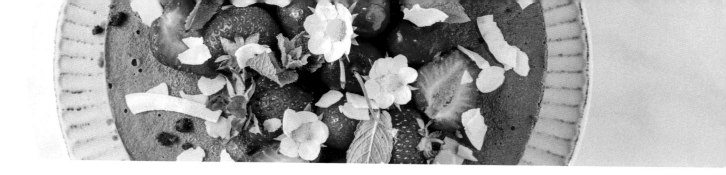

MIXED BERRY CHEESECAKE

This is one of my favorite deserts of ALL TIME to make during the holidays or for birthdays! It's so good, fairly easy to make and DELICIOUS! You've got to try it!

Crust

1 cup almonds
1/2 cup shredded coconut
15 medjool dates

Instructions:
Process almonds in food processor, then add coconut and dates and process until it becomes sticky. Press into a spring form cake pan.

Middle Layer

3 cups cashews (soaked for at least 4 hours, then drain water)
1 1/2 cups filtered water
1/2 cup coconut nectar
1 tsp vanilla bean powder or vanilla extract
Juice of 1 lemon (optional)

Instructions:
Blend all ingredients in a high speed blender until creamy. (If desired, you can substitute macadamia nuts for the cashews.) Pour into crust and place in freezer.

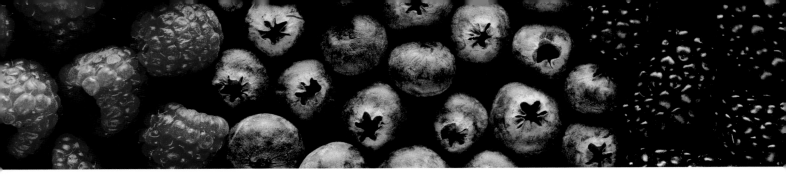

MIXED BERRY CHEESECAKE

Top Layer

1 cup mixed berries (or just strawberries as pictured above)
8 medjool dates
water (up to 1/2 cup)

Instructions:

Blend berries (you can use any berries or other fruit that you'd like!) and dates with 1/4 cup water. Add more water as necessary to form a thick sorbet texture. Pour berry mixture onto cake and return cake to freezer for 3 minutes prior to serving. Once ready to serve, decorate with berries, coconut flakes, edible flowers, etc.

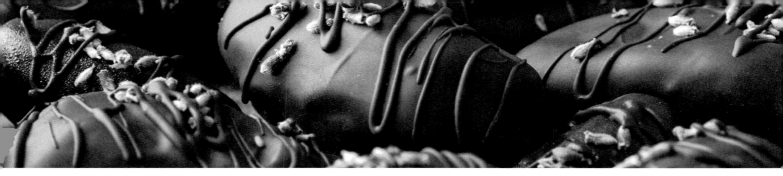

CHOCOLATE COVERED DATES

Chocolate Covered Dates

Dates
Almond Butter
Chocolate (I use the Hü Kitchen chocolate gems)

You will need:
Two bowls, one slightly larger than the other

Instructions:
Place 1 cup of water on stove to boil. Remove pit from dates. Place almond butter inside date. Place boiling water into the larger bowl. Grab the small bowl and place 1 cup of chocolates into bowl. Place the chocolate bowl on top of the boiling water bowl and let the chocolate melt. Stirring occasionally. Once chocolate has melted, place a fork into the date and roll it around in the chocolate. Use another fork to remove date from the fork. Place on parchment paper lined tray or Tupperware and place in the freezer. Repeat this process until down. Freeze for 10 min and they are ready to eat or then place them in the fridge.

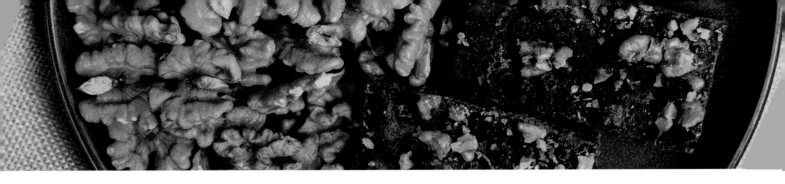

EASY RAW VEGAN BROWNIES

Easy Raw Vegan Brownies

2 cups raw walnuts
2 1/2 cups dates pitted, (if dry, soak in water for 10 minutes then drain)
3/4 cup cacao powder
2 Tbsp cacao nibs
1/4 tsp sea salt

TOPPINGS (optional)
walnuts
cacao nibs

Instructions:
Place 1 cup walnuts in food processor and process until finely ground. Add the cacao powder + salt and pulse to combine. Transfer to bowl and set aside.

Add the dates to the food processor and process until small bits remain. Remove and set aside.

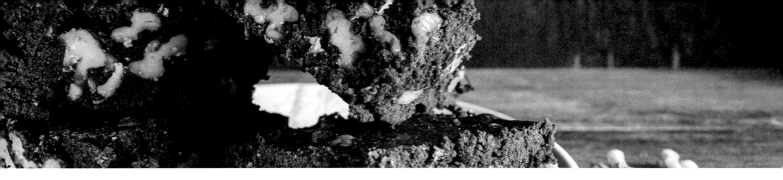

EASY RAW VEGAN BROWNIES

Add nut and cacao mixture back into food processor and while processing, drop small handfuls of the date pieces down into the food processor or blender spout.

Process until a dough consistency is achieved, adding more dates if the mixture does not hold together when squeezed in your hand. You may not use all the dates.

Add the brownie mixture to a small parchment lined 8x8 dish and before pressing, add remaining 1/2 cup roughly chopped walnuts (optional) and cacao nibs and toss to combine and evenly distribute. Then press down with hands until it is flat and firm. Place in freezer or fridge to chill for 10-15 minutes before cutting into 12 even squares.

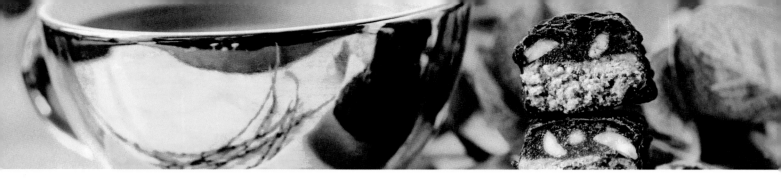

RAW VEGAN
SNICKERS BAR

These are one of my all time favorite things on planet earth!!! Serve these as desert after your next dinner party and your guests will fall in love!

Caramel Layer:

1 packed cup Medjool Dates
2 Tbsp Peanut Butter
1 tsp Vanilla Extract
1 tsp Maca
¼ tsp pink salt

Nougat Layer:

⅔ cup Oat Flour
¼ cup Date Caramel
⅓ cup the best peanuts you can find!

Chocolate (I use Hü Kitchen gems)

Instructions:

Remove the pits from the Dates and pack them (really pack them!) into 1 cup. Transfer the Dates to a larger bowl and cover with water. Soak the Dates for 1 hr or so in filtered water, depending on how dry they are.

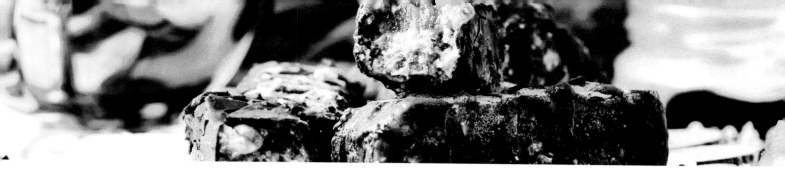

RAW VEGAN
SNICKERS BAR

If you do not have Oat Flour, make some by blending ⅔ cup of Quick or Rolled Oats in a Blender or food processor for 45-60 seconds until smooth and fluffy.

Drain any excess liquid off of the Dates (keep the water that they were soaking in!) Dates should be relatively moist, but not dripping and add them to a food processor or high speed blender with the remaining ingredients for the Caramel. Process until thick and smooth. Remove the Date Caramel from the food processor.

Add the Oat Flour back to the food processor or blender (no need to rinse) with ¼ cup of the Date Caramel and process until well incorporated. This should form a slightly sticky "dough" that will hold together when you pinch it.

Firmly and evenly press the Oat Flour Nougat into a container. Use a spatula to spread the remaining Date Caramel evenly over the Nougat, then sprinkle the Peanuts over the Caramel. Use your fingers to press the Peanuts into the Caramel layer, so they stick. Place this in the freezer for 1 hr.

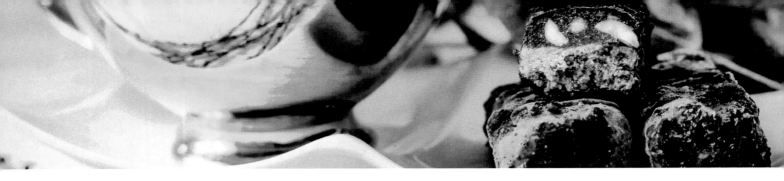

RAW VEGAN
SNICKERS BAR

Remove the frozen "filling" from its container, then use a sharp knife to cut it into bar-sized pieces or whatever shape you'd like (squares are nice too!)

Return these to the freezer while you melt your chocolate. Melt your Chocolate using either a double boiler or pan... Or... place boiling hot water into a bowl and add chocolate to a separate bowl. Place the bowl with chocolate on top of water bowl. Once the chocolate is 75% melted, stop and stir the mixture with a spatula until completely melted.

Moving quickly; place 1 candy bar into the bowl of melted Chocolate. Use two forks to "flip" the bar, until it is coated in chocolate on all sides. Remove from the melted Chocolate, letting any excess chocolate drip off. Then, place it onto a plate lined with parchment paper. Repeat with the remaining bars. Place the bars in the fridge for 5-10 minutes, to allow the Chocolate to harden. After 10 min remove from freezer and Viola! Raw Vegan snickers bars are ready to eat and they are INCREDIBLE!!!

Bars are best stored in the fridge. You can also place them in the freezer - just let the bars thaw for 5 or so minutes before eating. These bars are also SUPER yummy in vanilla nice cream! Just simply cut them up into small bites and stir into freshly made nice cream! YUMMMM!!!

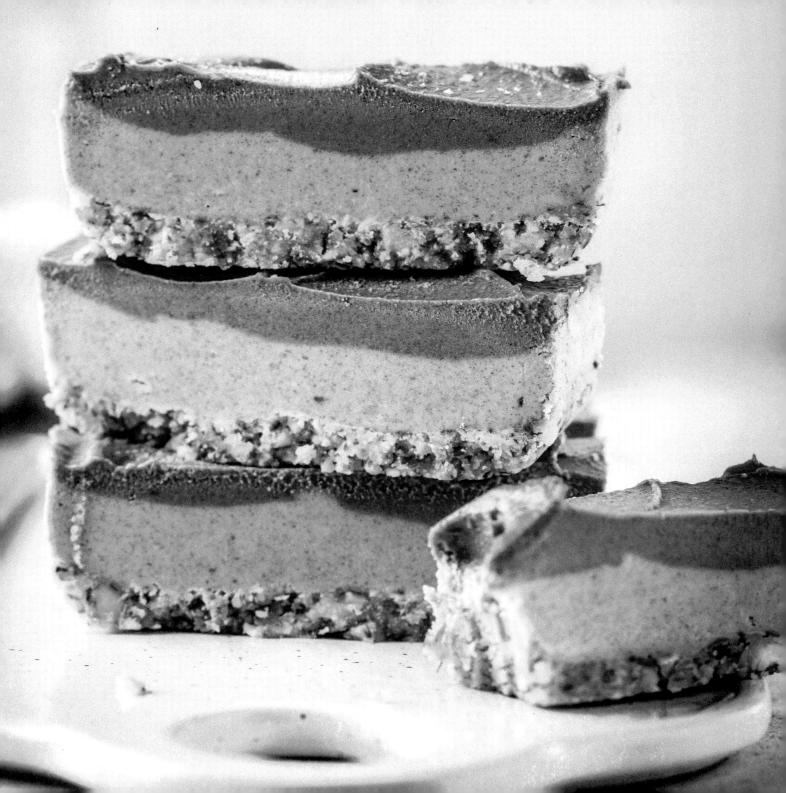

CHOCOLATE MULBERRY LAYERED DESSERT BARS

Ingredients:

Raw almonds (or any nuts of your choice!): ½ cup
Pitted dates: ¾ cup (12-14 dates total)
Raw cacao powder: 3 tbsp
Coconut oil: 2 tbsp (or you can also use 1/2 cup cashews)
Dried mulberries: ½ cup (soaked for at least 20 minutes)

Instructions:

1. Crust:

Blend ½ cup raw almonds, ½ cup pitted dates, 1 tbsp raw cacao powder, and a pinch of sea salt (optional) until crumbly. Press into the base of a lined pan.

2. First Layer:

Blend ½ cup dried soaked mulberries, 2 tbsp coconut oil or 1/2 cup cashews, and a few soaked dates (if desired) for sweetness until smooth. If using cashews – add water to blend. Spread on top of the crust.

3. Second Layer:

Blend ¼ cup pitted dates, ¼ cup cacao powder, 1 tbsp coconut oil, and a pinch of sea salt. (optional) Spread over the crust.

4. Chill in the fridge for at least 2 hours, slice, and enjoy!

This keeps the essence of the original recipe while simplifying the ingredients.

ABOUT THE AUTHOR

Jeannette Donofrio is the author of the best selling Raw Vegan Beauty Book, Raw Vegan Excuses Part One and Two, The Healing Powers of A Raw Vegan Diet, The Master Manifestor Journal, and many other ground-breaking books and courses in the plant-based and living foods community. She is extremely passionate about sharing her experience and knowledge of a fruit-based raw vegan lifestyle, which she has followed since 2011. Jeannette has naturally healed her cystic acne, chronic fatigue, migraine headaches, IBS, eczema, depression, chronic lung infections, chronic back and knee pain, and has lost over 60 lbs all by changing what she eats AND how she thinks!

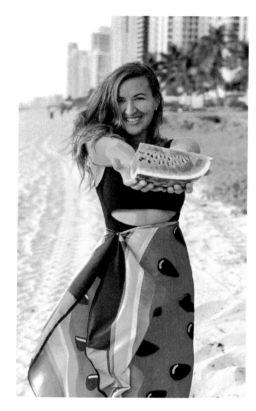

Since 2017, she has helped to coordinate The Woodstock Fruit Festival, the world's largest raw vegan retreat and now runs her own Raw Beauty Retreats in Miami, Florida! Jeannette is a former NYC Food and Beverage Business Consultant and is currently working towards opening Fruit Is Life, the world's FIRST fast-fruit restaurant!

Jeannette is dedicated to inspiring the world to eat more fruit instead of dead animal body parts and is committed to providing value through her free resources, podcast, courses, social media, and YouTube channel, where she posts daily content on fruit, healthy living, goal-achieving strategies, and more! Jeannette is one of the most authentic and trusted leaders in the raw vegan movement and goes by Ms.FitVegan on all social media platforms!

ADDITIONAL RESOURCES

· ·

Raw Vegan Excuses:
The Top 30 Reasons We Struggle
to Eat a Healthy Vegan Diet
(And The Solutions)

The Raw Vegan Beauty Book:
All Natural Beauty Secret | Tips
and Tricks That Actually Work!

**The Healing Powers of
A Raw Vegan Diet!**
100 Life Changing Testimonials of
What raw Foods Can Do!

**The Master Manifestor
Journal:**
A Proven Tool for Getting Things
Accomplished and Manifesting
Miracles in Your Life!

Raw Vegan Excuses Part II:
The Last of The Excuses!

Gratitude Journal:
90-Days Of Practice

All Available On Amazon Now!

Where To Go From Here!

I know it seems hard to be healthy sometimes, but never forget that it's also extremely hard to be overweight, uncomfortable, sick and in pain.

The good news is that you get to **CHOOSE YOUR HARD!**

I hope and pray that this book inspires you to choose the hard work that it takes to be healthy. It's worth it!

Let's connect and stay on a healthy raw vegan lifestyle TOGETHER!

www.MsFitVegan.com

You can find me on social media:

Instagram: @Ms.FitVegan

YouTube: Ms.FitVegan

My FREE Private Facebook Group: Misfit Mondays

TikTok: @MsFitVegan

Apple Podcast + Spotify: The MsFitVegan Podcast

You can check out my VIVP (very important vegan person)
Private Community at www.MisfitMondays.com

**Want to find out more information about my next
6-Week Food Addiction Freedom Course?**

Send me an email with the words "I Am Ready" in the subject
and I will send you all the details!

If you have ANY questions about this book or ANYTHING at all,
do not hesitate to reach out!

My personal email address is JD@MsFitVegan.com

Thank you again for investing in this book and in YOURSELF!

#EatFruitBeCute

Jeannette

THANK YOU!

· ·

I hope by receiving this book it inspires you to try something new and maybe even replace an unhealthy favorite with one of these recipes.

Thank you for investing in this book!

Jeannette Donofrio | @Ms.FitVegan

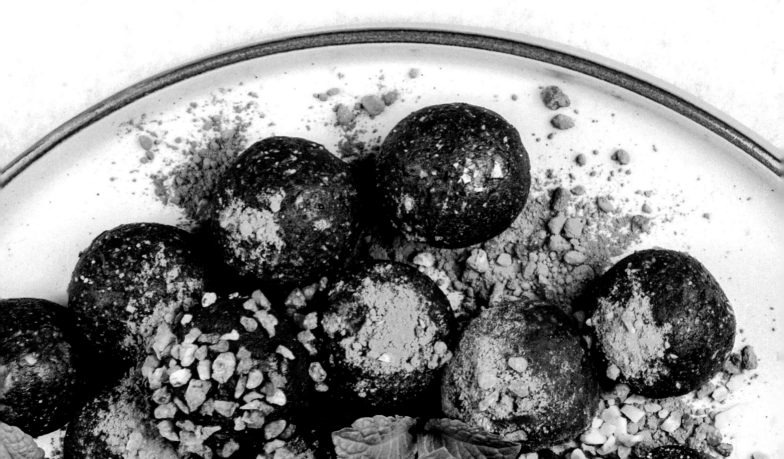

Made in the USA
Las Vegas, NV
06 June 2025

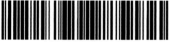

23262274R00076